Diary of an ADHD Mum

Diary of an ADHD Mum

Learning to live, love & laugh
parenting a child with ADHD

Susy O'Hare

First published in 2017 as Saving Sarah; learning to live, love & laugh with ADHD Second addition 2019 Diary of an ADHD Mum; learning to live, love & laugh parenting a child with ADHD by Susy O'Hare.
All rights reserved. Printed in the USA.

Published by Author Academy Elite, P.O. Box 43, Powell, OH 430065
www.authoracademyelite.com

Library of congress cataloguing: 2019914151

Softcover: 978-1-64085-929-6
Hardcover: 978-1-64085-930-2
E-book: 978-1-64085-931-9

Available in hardcover, softcover, e-book, and audiobook

Cover photos Bronnie Joel Photography

To protect the privacy of the people in the book, some names have been changed to protect their identities.

For Seren, I love you more than all the stars.

Author's note

The information, including but not limited to, text, graphics, images and any other material contained in this book is purely for informational purposes and does not purport to be comprehensive. We do not give any warranty that the information is free from error or suitable for your purposes. You should carefully evaluate the accuracy, completeness and relevance of any information.

The purpose of this book is to share our journey with other parents. I haven't got a degree in psychology or psychiatry; I'm not a pediatrician or a naturopath, but what I do have is experience, so I hope that our experiences can help other parents and children. I have read countless books on ADHD; I have watched numerous experts talk about how the brain works, the lack of dopamine, the difference in the way transmitters speak to each other and how ADHD has comorbid symptoms such as Oppositional Defiance Disorder, tics and dyslexia, etc. There are many experts all over the planet with their theories, diets, pills, ideas, concepts and medications. This is just our story, our journey and my opinions, feelings and thoughts.

However, it's important to mention that our journey is not intended to be a substitute for professional medical or psychological advice, diagnosis or treatment and no responsibility is accepted for any loss arising from reliance on it. You should never disregard professional medical or psychological advice or delay seeking assistance and advice from such professionals because of something you have read in this book. You should never cease medication because of any of the information in this book. We strongly advise that you consult a medical health professional before relying on any information contained in this book.

With love & light
Susy x

Note to the reader

My name is Susy, and my intention is to help you step out of a lens of fear, and step into a lens of love. As you begin this journey, you can be thrown into a tsunami of chaos. You will have many different fears placed upon you from experts, teachers, friends, family and society. I am here to lovingly remind you that all will be well, my friend. If you work on connecting with yourself and your child, and always come back to your heart and intuition, your child will begin to thrive (and so will you).

It's been two years since I first published my book and three years since I wrote it. Initially, I called it Saving Sarah, but I felt that the dairy of an ADHD mum was more suited, as that's precisely what this book is about. I'm now living free of fear sharing our story, so I changed the name from Sarah to my daughter's real name, Seren. Her name means Star in Welsh and what a star this girl has become. She has grown into her name and I couldn't be more proud of her. I also decided to change my pen name, Susy Parker, to my real name, Susy O'Hare. I want to be as honest, open and vulnerable as I can. I believe if we're going to make a change in this world, we need to be as authentic as possible. We must be brave and allow ourselves to be truly seen.

I also wanted to republish my book as when it was first published; I was feeling overwhelmed, scared and heavy about sharing our story. I didn't give this book what it deserved. I didn't go out and meet the people and share my story to those who needed to hear my words. Frightened, worried and lacking in confidence, my book was published out to the world, but I went within. I went through somewhat of a breakdown, which ultimately became my breakthrough. I stepped bravely into the work of un-becoming everything that I thought I was supposed to be and finally found myself. I began to heal and work through my deepest, darkest pain. It was here that I found myself, and it was the start of Seren becoming who she was supposed to be in this life, free of limiting labels and now thriving as her beautiful self.

Seren has just turned twelve years old and what a ride it's been! She isn't medicated anymore and hasn't been since she was eight years old. She is doing incredibly well at school, is a talented acrobat, horse rider and self-taught contortionist. She plays guitar in a band and is determined to only show up in this world as herself, not who others want her to be. Seren is thriving, has friends and is the happiest, most resilient kid ever! However, this doesn't mean this ride is easy. Seren is fiercely headstrong, independent, spirited, determined and at times still challenging to parent. These kids don't come with a set of instructions, so as I navigate these uncharted waters, I continue to work on myself, my healing and my happiness as it is from this place, I can hold space for my daughter.

Along the way, I was diagnosed with ADHD and PMDD. I went on a two-year journey of self-discovery, deep healing and awakening, which I will be sharing more in my next book. I believe wholeheartedly that to heal our children, it must begin with us first and foremost. Once I started to get out of the victim mentality and to see that she was in my life for a reason, I could begin to see the gift within the darkness. I was able to finally allow myself to crack wide open and begin a new journey of self-discovery for myself, my family and for Seren.

I want you to begin this journey with trust, compassion and love. I want you to be guided by your intuition and go to the places that often feel the most uncomfortable. There will be so many lessons along the way that you must endure but always come back to your values and your truth. You will be given so much information on this journey, many of it will not be the truth, so always come back to that beautiful intuition of yours. Do what feels right in your soul and your heart, and you will always be led by love.

Susy x

Introduction

Life is crazy, especially when you have three little kids and one comes with a set of interesting differences. It can certainly make life a little more complicated!

I have found that writing this book has been hugely cathartic. It has helped our situation enormously, as all my thoughts and feelings were whirling around inside my head. To be able to put pen to paper has allowed me to organise these thoughts and to become a better parent to Seren. It also helped me finally make peace with the ADHD diagnosis.

I would get up every morning at 5.00 am to write this book, which would give me a couple of 'quiet' hours before the children got up. One particular morning, Seren got up really early and found me at the kitchen table sitting in the darkness typing away at my computer.

'What are you doing, Mummy?' she asked.

'I'm writing my book, the one to help other parents and children who are experiencing something similar to us. There could be another family whose child has ADHD, and reading this book may help them in some way. It may help the child too,' I replied.

Seren thought for a while and then said, 'I think the doctors don't know what they are doing. Children are really scared, and the doctors don't know what the children are actually capable of. When they know, they will see that they are beautiful children and don't need medication.'

What she said that morning made me cry. We had spent the last eighteen months feeling so hard done by, and as a family we felt emotionally drained from the whole experience. We were scared, lost and frightened as we found ourselves in a whirlwind of diagnoses.

To us, it felt like Seren had been giving us a hard time. But what she said that day made me realise that she hadn't been giving us a hard time, she had been having a hard time.

For the first time, I could see the huge impact all this had on Seren, and I came to learn that it wasn't just about us – it was about Seren. She was a little girl who had been just as scared, lost and frightened as us, but she didn't have the words to tell us, so instead her behaviour did the talking.

A psychologist diagnosed Seren with ADHD and anxiety when she was just six years old. This was then confirmed by a pediatrician one week before her seventh birthday. Months later, a second pediatrician diagnosed Seren with ADHD and Oppositional Defiance Disorder.

As a mum, it almost broke me as I watched my daughter, my first born, my beautiful baby girl, spiral out of control. I had no idea how to stop it; it was like a relentless fire burning through our home destroying everything in its wake.

We tried different types of medication, various parenting styles, and we listened to all the conflicting medical advice about how to 'fix' our daughter. We spent thousands of dollars, until one day – broken, depressed and at rock bottom – I found my strength and realised that I had to fix it.

I had to make everything right.

The day that we stepped away from all the advice, the drugs, the tests, the opinions and the labels was the day that we saved our family. It was the day that I saved my sanity. More importantly, it's the day that we saved Seren.

Throughout this book, I share the personal diary I wrote during the eighteen-month period, starting when Seren was diagnosed with ADHD.

I am not on a quest to stop parents medicating their children, and I am not on a mission to belittle the medical profession. I want to empower parents to make the right choices to help themselves and to help their children thrive.

I have tried to draw on positives as I have been writing this book, as I believe that there are positives in every situation in life, even if we can't see them straightaway sometimes. For me, the positive through all of this was spending more time with Seren.

At the time, she drove me crazy and just being with her would send my head into a spin. However, while this journey took me to the darkest depths, it also gave me a better, healthier, happier relationship with Seren.

Unfortunately, this wouldn't become apparent until the very end of the journey.

I am sharing Seren's story to let other parents know that there can be another way and that miracles do happen, because a miracle happened to us.

ADHD – it's just a different way to be.

In a Blanket of Stars

This book is dedicated to you my love
My wonderful little star
I'm so proud of you for what you've achieved
And how amazing you really are

I hope one day the dark memories fade
And you only remember the light
Many more memories that we can make
Your future now shines so bright

We hit rock bottom and held hands as we fell
Then we held each other tight
I wrapped you up in a blanket of stars
And together we followed the light

I hope one day when you read this book
You won't be cross with me
And you'll realise my darling, why I did it
To help other parents just like me

Because ADHD is really a gift
And children should feel really proud
It shouldn't need hiding or treating with drugs
Just to make them blend into the crowd

So for now I will finish my ode to you
My beautiful shining star
Thank you for travelling this journey with me
And well done for coming so far

And if anything else should come your way
I will wrap you in a blanket of stars
I will love you until the end of the Earth,
Jupiter, Neptune and Mars.

Mummy x

Chapter One

There is no such thing as normal

They say that you can always tell that your child is different. We knew that Seren was different when she was a baby – her determination, fearless attitude and her amazing ability to bounce the living day lights out of her baby rocker with her foot, way before she could even lift her head!

Six weeks after Karl and I got married, Seren was conceived and I was the happiest I had ever been.

My parents separated when I was fourteen. Their marriage had always been tempestuous – fighting and arguing was all I had ever known. We lived in a beautiful home in the country and had wonderful holidays; however, behind closed doors, it was a very different story.

My mother was an alcoholic, although she would never admit it. She was on a mission to change the world, one letter at a time. It seemed like she was always 'fighting' someone – a neighbour, the council, the government, and my dad. She was a councillor in the local village and spent most days sending letters to people, trying to change things about the village. She would also drink whisky (in a teacup, pretending she was drinking tea), and she would do all this while lost in a hazy mist of silk-cut cigarette smoke! I do have some fond memories of her baking and cooking delicious meals, wearing beautiful dresses, smelling of wonderful perfume and dancing and singing in the living room. But those happy memories faded many years ago, as sadly I haven't had a relationship with my mother for almost twenty-five years.

I sometimes wonder how the hell it all happened? How could she not have held my babies, been there for me during the dark times, and held my hand and laughed with me during the happy times. When my parents divorced, I made the decision to live with my dad and unfortunately mother could never forgive me for this. Even though I have come to terms with it, it will always be a painful ache in my heart.

My past defined me for a long time, and even now it makes me feel uncomfortable when remembering those times. I desperately wanted to be 'normal', to fit in, to be liked, to be accepted.

I left school, and home, at the age of fifteen. My dad also remarried when I was fifteen. I call his new wife, Karen, my 'mum', even though she isn't my birth mother – she has been the only real mum that I have had. I am so grateful to her for mothering me, as I'm sure I tested her at times

So here I was, aged twenty-nine, married to the love of my life and pregnant with my first baby. We were living in a little village on the Wirral, northwest England, in an old Victorian flat that we had renovated over the last twelve months. Karl had recently started his own business and, with a new baby, we found ourselves in unfamiliar territory. However, we were happy and in love and life felt great. We were both looking forward to this next stage in our lives.

We'd been together for seven years and I had been desperate to start a family as soon as we could. I think I had been broody for about ten years! I started to become addicted to watching baby TV programs, and thought constantly about what it would feel like to have a baby. All our friends were starting to have babies; in fact, we were nearly completely surrounded by bumps and babies. Most of our friends had married over the last two years and I loved being a part of this next stage.

As luck would have it, my path to pregnancy was a smooth one. I was so lucky, managing to get pregnant six weeks after we got married.

I remember for my 30th birthday, Karl bought me a puppy (Chip). I was so broody but Karl tried to convince me that it wasn't the right time for a baby. He had recently started his own business and money was tight, so he felt we needed to wait. He thought that a puppy would be the perfect distraction, but I had other ideas ...

We had a little home and some old furniture that we bought from the second-hand shop. We had done everything we could to set up a home and make it the perfect setting for our growing family. I had read every baby book and watched every baby program, and I felt so ready for this exciting new chapter.

Everything was starting to feel normal and I loved this feeling. I wondered if this was how everyone else felt. Married – check, pregnant – check, in love – check.

However, these wonderful feelings only started after I became pregnant. For twelve months before the pregnancy, life had been pretty crazy! I will talk more later about how I was feeling during this time in my life, but the months before I conceived Seren definitely weren't normal.

Being married and pregnant made me feel great. I had done it, against all the odds of growing up with my parents fighting, my mother drinking, and lots more craziness that would take me another book to write, here I was … happily married and pregnant. But there was more craziness to come, that's for sure.

If there is one thing that I have learnt over the last ten years – there is no such thing as 'normal'.

Seren's early years

Seren was our first child and we loved her with everything we had. She was the first grandchild for the family and everyone adored her.

My two friends and myself had daughters within weeks of each other, and we started attending baby classes together. Baby sensory, rhythm time, baby signing, baby swimming, dates in the park – I was hooked! I had never noticed this happy 'baby world' before. No-one had ever spoken of it and it totally blew my mind! Breastfeeding, sling wearing, comfy-pants living, baby-book reading, I felt like it was my calling in life.

I started to notice early on – probably at around six months old – that Seren was quite 'spirited'. She was curious, determined and she knew her mind, even at such a tender age.

When Seren was thirteen months old, my goddaughter who was three at the time came for a play date. I remember Seren not letting her play with anything, screeching at her every time she played with her toys and even biting her. I know this is entirely normal, but as the years passed this trend was here to stay.

Biting children, being asked to leave baby classes, refusing to sit in the car seat, refusing to sit in her buggy, tearing books to shreds, drawing on the walls and furniture, climbing, tantrums – it was never-ending. I found Seren so hard to manage that we didn't even think about having another baby for four years after she was born.

Seren ran everywhere, and when she wasn't running, she was hiding. There were so many times that I was panic-stricken, running deliriously around a shop screaming, 'I've lost my daughter'. Almost every time, she was hiding underneath a bed or hiding in a rack of clothes or behind a mannequin. I thought I was going to go mad – this was all before Seren was two years old!

Our only resort was to use the 'naughty step'. The naughty-step memories give me shudders, as I now realise that I was just reinforcing the fact that Seren was 'naughty'. However, at the time, it was the only thing I had; I didn't know any other option.

Even at this young age, shopping was always hard with Seren. I used to be in awe of my friend who took her four-year-old and two-year-old food shopping every Friday. I always thought maybe I was doing something wrong.

Seren was able to bring pandemonium to a shop within minutes – when she was only two! She would always grab the clothes as we would pass the racks of cute dresses. They would all crash to the floor, and while I would be gathering them together, Seren would be grabbing more items of clothes and pulling them to the floor. It always amazed me how she did this when she was only a toddler, with little toddler arms, and was strapped into her buggy – a child genius, surely.

I recall a time when some very prestigious shops opened in a new centre in Liverpool, called 'Liverpool One'. I wasn't one for shopping in designer stores, but this particular day I thought I would have a quick peep. Seren was about three and was as curious and callous as ever.

The shop assistant, with her perfectly pressed clothes and beautiful smile, asked me if I would like any help. I suddenly felt a little intimidated as I realised that I was in my scruffy workout attire. I opened my mouth and was just about to say, 'I'm fine, thank you. I'm just browsing', when the mannequin, that was as beautifully dressed as the shop assistant, came falling to the floor with a crash! Clothes, jewellery and handbags were flying everywhere like a trapeze artist's routine gone wrong, and among the craziness was Seren.

Now here is the difference – many kids at this age would have some remorse. They may run and hide behind their parent's legs in total embarrassment. They might mutter out a quick, 'Sorry Mummy', but not Seren. She was completely and utterly unaware of the havoc that she had caused. And before I could grab her, she was pulling clothes from the hangers, or pulling more jewellery off the arm of the mannequin (which was what got us into this mess in the beginning)!

Seren seemed to have zero empathy for any chaos she had caused. If she had bitten a child – 'so what'; coloured all Mummy's white leather chairs pink – 'it wasn't me'; or ran across the road as a lorry was passing – 'it wasn't my fault'. There was no empathy, no remorse, no apologies and often no tears. It was all very strange and hard to deal with as a first-time mummy.

When your toddler utters those words, 'Sorry Mummy', you can often find yourself melting in their cuteness. A normal response would be, 'It isn't that bad', 'It will wash', 'We can paint it', and the favourite, 'No-one got hurt'. But Seren didn't have that ability to make me feel like that. She would make me even madder, and I could feel steam coming out of my ears!

When Seren started nursery, age three, I was called in at regular intervals as Seren had bitten various children. This happened a lot and it was starting to become quite normal. I remember one of the mums pulling me aside after Seren had bitten her little girl and informing me that she was taking her child to have a tetanus shot. I did think it was a little extreme and apologised profusely, but little did I know that there were going to be many of these conversations with parents in the coming years. However, they would get worse and harder to deal with.

When Seren was four years old, her teacher called me in to talk about the fact that Seren wasn't showing any empathy. She would upset her friends and then walk off, not realising that she had upset them. I brushed this off completely and wondered how silly it was to talk about a four-year-old having empathy.

Now, after having two other children, I realise that empathy is something that you are born with. At the time of writing this, even my two-year-old has empathy and will say sorry to his older sister if he hurts her (ok, so not all the time, but it's there).

Play dates were difficult, there was always fighting, crying, arguing, biting, hitting and general chaos whenever we were there. However, as Seren was my first child, I thought this was how kids were supposed to be. However, as time passed, we started noticing big differences between our friend's children and Seren. We were now starting to question our parenting. Was it something that we were doing wrong?

Seren would never listen; she would never do as she was told. She was overly emotional, hyperactive and defiant. We really wanted to have another baby, all of our friends were having baby number two, and I wanted this too. If I'm honest we found Seren such a handful that I was worried how I would cope with another baby – I felt like I could hardly cope with one! We figured that Seren would be Seren whether we had another baby or not, so just after Seren's third birthday, we decided to try for another baby.

We conceived Daisy on a weekend trip away to Rome to celebrate our fourth wedding anniversary. I remember feeling so elated after I gave birth to Daisy that, I think, Seren's behaviour didn't affect me as much for a short time. I was in a happy bubble of bliss with two beautiful girls and I felt like the luckiest woman alive!

Seren's and Daisy's births

Daisy was born at home in a birthing pool, using nothing else other than homeopathy, essential oils, and HypnoBirthing.

I also used HypnoBirthing with the birth of Seren; however, it was a much longer birth (twenty-one hours) that had the usual hospital interventions – sweeps, waters broken, and the syntocin drip to bring on the labour. After I had the syntocin drip, the contractions came fast and constant, and I decided to have an epidural, which then slowed the labour down and then I needed assistance to birth Seren. She was in the back-to-back position, so the doctor gave her a manual rotation. I am sure this wasn't the birth that Seren was expecting, and neither was I.

Nevertheless, with the Carpenters playing and my stepmum, Karen, and Karl there, I still remember it as a beautiful birth. I had felt like I was in control the whole time, but there had been lots of 'helping hands' and drugs, and I was convinced that labour didn't have to be like that. Thanks to the HypnoBirthing method, I was able to stay calm, focused and empowered during Seren's birth.

HypnoBirthing teaches women to stay calm during labour. Different words are also used. For example, in HypnoBirthing we call a contraction a 'surge'. During the surge you use the breath, music and visualisations to stay calm and focused. It's a way of taking birth right back to basics – you walk, you breathe, and often the babies are born in water. I practised this method throughout Seren's birth, and although I still opted for an epidural towards the end of my labour, I felt in control the whole time. Overall, I still view Seren's birth experience as a positive one.

A year after having Seren, I qualified to become a HypnoBirthing practitioner and then taught numerous women to achieve calmer births, often without medication. I always felt that the reason I took drugs with Seren's birth was because they were available. I was in hospital and that's what you did, that's how birth was – it was painful and drugs took away or helped with the pain.

During my HypnoBirthing classes, I would show a video of a Hypno- Birth to the parents to be. These videos showed women in labour being really calm, breathing through their surges and even talking and laughing between surges – all of the women were so calm that they didn't need medication.

When I became pregnant with Daisy, I decided to have her at home as I felt that this would be the perfect place to have my baby. I practised daily hypnosis, relaxation and breathing – and if my labour wasn't progressing I could walk up and down the stairs and have a hot bath, just like the 'old days'.

Daisy's birth is without a doubt one of the most powerful, amazing experiences of my life. It sounds so silly when I say this, but I felt so connected to nature that day. I felt like Mother Earth was with me every step of the way, holding my hand. From walking through the woods and leaning on a tree during my contractions, and then Daisy being born in the warm water in the stillness of the night – it was magical.

I was so passionate about helping other women achieve this type of birth that I decided to film the birth. I had no idea that Daisy's birth was going to be like that; I don't think I thought I was capable of achieving something so natural, calm and serene. I was the girl who would scream the house down if I stubbed my toe!

I shared Daisy's birth with another HypnoBirthing practitioner who was also a midwife. She contacted me straight after she watched it and asked me if I would talk to a group of midwives at a seminar in Liverpool. I was really nervous, but I went along, holding a six-week-old Daisy, and talked to forty midwives and then showed them the birth. Most of them had never seen a birth like it! Then one of the UK's top midwives asked me if she could have a copy of the birth. She was giving a talk in Japan to ninety midwives and wanted to show them how birth could be. She used to consult with the government on their practices, so it was a big deal that she wanted to show them Daisy's birth.

My inbox became full of requests for Daisy's birth. Midwives told me that they had never seen anything like it. Even my midwife said that she had never witnessed a calm birth like that before in her twenty-five years of being a midwife. Daisy's birth has been watched over 200,000 times, and people from all over the world have emailed me to thank me for sharing it. I even bumped into a HypnoBirthing practitioner at Seren's school recently. She recognised me calling Daisy and then came over to talk to me. She told me that she had been showing Daisy's birth to all her HypnoBirthing mums for the last four years here in Perth – I couldn't believe it! Little Daisy's birth at home in a birthing pool in Wales was being used on the other side of the world.

I draw a lot of similarities to HypnoBirthing with our ADHD journey with Seren. We listened to the experts, we took the drugs, and then we learnt that there was a different path. So with one foot in front of the other, not really knowing which direction we were heading, we chose a different route.

Life before HypnoBirthing

For four years before I conceived Seren, I had worked in television and radio and absolutely loved it. It was my dream to work in television, after appearing on TV when I was younger. I landed my perfect job working for ITV in London, and Karl and I spent twelve months living in the 'big smoke'. He had recently had a promotion and I was now working at the ITV studios on the Thames, however, there was only one problem. I am not a city girl and I realised this soon after I arrived. A year later, we moved back to our hometown and Karl started his own business.

I landed a new TV job but it was a four-hour trip to work and back every day, plus a sixty-hour working week on top. I knew this wasn't what I was destined to do, at now twenty-nine years of age. I was desperate to become a mum, so after my contract finished I didn't return to TV.

Shortly after we got married, I qualified to become a holistic therapist, and then after Seren was born, as I mentioned before, I qualified to become a HypnoBirthing practitioner. I wanted to slow things down and try a new career path – something that I could do from home with a baby. Hypno-Birthing seemed perfect.

Over the years I have been many things – a pot washer, a waitress, a bartender, a sales person, a marketing researcher, a radio presenter, a TV assistant producer, a PA, a HypnoBirthing practitioner, a holistic therapist, a Pilates teacher and now an author (although this one has surprised me the most). I used to feel embarrassed that I tried my hand at so many different career paths. I sometimes felt like I was just flitting from one thing to another.

If I am honest, my single most important goal was always to be a mum. Everything I was doing before that was just 'paying the bills' and giving me some sort of normality, helping me in some way to finally find my destiny in life. I always knew that I wanted to have children and be a stay-at-home mum, so for this to finally be happening was a dream come true.

Looking back, I can see why this journey with Seren almost broke me. I felt that I was failing – failing as a mother and failing in my chosen path in life. Only during this process with Seren did it become apparent to me why I had always chopped and changed my way through both my twenties and thirties. Only during this experience have I realised that this journey hasn't been my downfall. It was simply a stepping-stone to reach my destiny, which was to help Seren discover who she was, not who society wanted her to be.

Flynn's birth

Two years after giving birth to Daisy, I filmed my third child's birth. Flynn's birth was also at home – same setting, same birth pool, same vibe as Daisy's birth.

Daisy's birth was a breeze. It was a textbook delivery. Flynn, however, had other ideas. His birth was more of a comedy sketch. He was almost even born in the toilet! I think, being a boy, he wanted a more exciting birth other than being born in a Zen birthing pool. It makes me laugh thinking about it, as Seren has blurted this out to so many people at the most inappropriate times. I remember one morning as we were crossing the road to Seren's school, she blurted out to one of the dads, 'My brother was born in the toilet'. The dad looked a bit embarrassed but weirdly we ended up having a great conversation about natural childbirth and how the caesarean rate is increasing each year.

Too much cortisol?

I have learnt so much over the last ten years since I conceived Seren, and I have changed so much as a person.

At the time of conceiving Seren, I was stressed, depressed and anxious. I had recently moved, recently changed career paths but still didn't know which direction I was heading. And due to certain circumstances, which I will come to later, I was suffering from PTSD and anxiety, and I am convinced that Seren was created with way too much cortisol (the stress hormone)!

We are told that drugs, cigarette smoke and alcohol are bad for our babies. We are told that blue cheese and brie are a no-no, but no-one really talks about stress! And I have always wondered whether my anxiety before I conceived, and Seren's birth, affected the way she has been in her life. Unfortunately, I will never know, no-one can say, but I honestly feel that the stress I experienced leading up to conceiving her impacted on her chemical makeup. Sure, I created her with pure love. She was desperately wanted, and I always felt that Seren saved me, having a baby was what I yearned for, for so long. So maybe the stress I was feeling altered her chemical makeup and caused her to act differently to other children. Maybe when I gave birth to her, the stress I felt affected her. Of course I will never be sure; however, these thoughts have plagued me.

Having serious doubts

Seren had been with me almost full-time before Daisy was born, and family and friends felt that this could have caused the problem – Seren wasn't used to sharing me.

I started to doubt myself and my parenting skills. I considered that maybe everyone else was doing it better and that maybe Seren would have been better at day care. Maybe I hadn't played enough with her, maybe we should have done more craft, more reading, had more adventures. We had done lots of things together, but everything was hard with Seren, everything was a challenge.

I loved baking, and I had baked with my grandma and my nana from a very young age. But when I was baking with Seren, with our matching pink polka dot pinnys on, our matching pink bowls and eggs at the ready, it would very quickly turn into chaos. She would grab, pinch, steal, not let go ... it was hard. Baking would turn into, 'Seren no', 'Seren, don't throw the eggs', 'Seren, don't throw the flour', 'Seren, mind your fingers that is a sharp blade', 'Seren, be careful the oven is hot', 'Seren, no, please don't feed the chocolate to the dog'! It was a nightmare and very stressful, and we were only trying to make a few bloody chocolate cupcakes!

Seren seemed to crave attention, and it didn't matter whether it was good or bad attention, as long as the focus was on her. She didn't enjoy make-believe play, didn't enjoy reading, and didn't ever play by herself, which was draining as a mum. And of course she didn't play very well with other children because she wasn't able to share, which would make play times very difficult.

Seren once lined up all her Barbie dolls face down on the floor. When Karl asked her what they were doing, she told him, 'They are all dead, Daddy'. We laughed at the time, and it still makes me giggle at the ridiculousness of it, but that pretty much summed up Seren's imaginative play!

Over the years I have been amazed while watching other children play imaginative play, which I remember doing myself as a child. I could play for hours and hours with nothing other than my imagination. I didn't even have anything in front of me, no toys, no objects, but I would play 'mummy and daddy' by myself for hours in the garden. I would make the dinner, strip the beds, take the dog for a walk ... I can see it now – I loved that game. However, I never saw Seren doing anything like this.

And it wasn't just the fact that Seren didn't seem to play like other children. Her behaviour was so bad at times that we couldn't get her to obey a simple instruction. From the minute she woke up she often refused to get dressed, eat her breakfast, let me do her hair or put on her school shoes. She would continually run off on the way to school, and I would be running after her, screaming, 'Seren stop, Seren stop'. She would run across the road without hesitation, and she'd be so crazy and hyper at times that she was unable to look me in the eye or focus on my face as I tried to speak to her.

Dinner times were extremely difficult. She refused to eat the food that I had made for her, she would be up and down 100 times or more at the dinner table, and then she'd refuse to tidy up her toys or get in the bath. Everything we asked her to do would be answered with 'no', and if we tried to tell her off she would very quickly start screaming and shouting at us.

Time for school

The day finally came when Seren was to start full-time school. She was only four years old. Phew, I had made it! I had reached the milestone. I couldn't wait for the break where I could just sit and have a cup of tea and relax – well relax as much as I could with a newborn.

11

I feel it's important to mention here that Seren turned four only two weeks before she started full-time school. If she had been born fourteen days later, she wouldn't have started school until the age of five. I don't think we appreciate the difference in a year, and how this can affect children's learning and behaviours. Recent studies are proving that this is the case and that the youngest children in the class can often be diagnosed with ADHD and medicated more frequently than their friends who are older. This research is conclusive all over the world and the final study on this was completed at the end of 2016.[1]

Seren's first day at school was an exciting one in our household. She seemed fine about the fact that she was about to go to school. She had been going to the nursery at the school since she was three years old. Here she had met a little girl called Betsy, and although there had been an incident where she had bitten Betsy, they seemed to be good little buddies.

I will always remember the first day of school for Seren; she and Betsy jumped up and down in pure excitement. In true Seren fashion, she had posed her usual pose when I took her picture outside school that morning – hand on hip, leg pointed out to the side. Even at four years old, she had the confidence and demeanour of someone much older than her years.

I remember feeling quite emotional when Seren started school that day. She was so excited and ran confidently into school after saying goodbye to us. I took some photos outside the school of her and Betsy and walked home with a sleeping Daisy in the pram.

We had managed to spend the summer together as a family and I was really glad for that time, all of us together. Karl was unable to take any time off when Seren was born, but he did work from home so it's not like he wasn't around. When Daisy was born, he was only able to take two weeks off, so it was wonderful to have him at home with me, Seren and Daisy during the summer holidays.

Seren's first day of school went really well. I remember her coming home and crashing out on the sofa. She didn't even take her coat off; she just collapsed in a heap. That night was pretty easy too – dinner, bath and bed. I liked this new world. This new Seren who had been stimulated and worn out all day was much easier to manage. Life was great!

All seemed to be going well, so far so good. I felt relieved ...

However, only a few weeks later, there was an incident when Karl went to collect her from school as a surprise. She wasn't expecting Karl, as I usually picked her up, so she screamed for me and refused to get into the car. She ran off down the road, and Karl chased after her, picking her up when he caught up to her down the road. Seren was screaming, physically kicking and punching him as he tried to hold her.

Karl had wanted to surprise her, yet he found himself almost in tears as he fought with Seren just to get her in the car. He arrived home and looked traumatised, wondering, 'How can she act like that? What am I supposed to do?'

Karl told me that the whole time he was driving home from school, Seren was screaming, 'Let me out, let me out now', while kicking the back of his car seat. Seren's behaviour was so out of control and so outlandish. What was happening? *Why was she acting this way and what the hell could we do to make it stop?*

Asking for parenting methods

When the naughty step wasn't working anymore, I found myself asking friends and family what type of parenting methods they were using, or had been using, with their children. Seren was getting wise to the fact that I was just making the naughty step up as I went along. 'That's not even a naughty step, it's a rock,' Seren would scream. I would then scream back, 'No it's not, it's a naughty step'. She was quite aware that the rock next to the elephant enclosure at the zoo was not a 'naughty step', and it was starting to make a mockery out of my parenting style.

Karl's uncle had older children who, at the time, were nine and eleven years old. They are the best-behaved kids that I have probably ever met. Ruby and Rex came to play at our house from time to time and they would sometimes stay for a sleepover. They were as good as gold – polite, friendly, happy and helpful children. Ruby played with Seren, and Rex would play and coo over Daisy for hours.

I remember asking Karl's Auntie Carol one day how she parented Rex and Ruby, as they were both so well behaved. She insisted that they weren't like that at home and that she didn't know what she was doing either. She went on to tell me about one thing that had worked, and that was the 'pasta in the jar' method – she had made it up herself, but she said it worked a treat.

Carol went on to tell me that she would take some dried pasta and put it in an empty jam jar. Every time they were naughty, or didn't do as they are told, she would take some pasta out of the jar. If they did something good, then the pasta would go back into the jar. She suggested starting it on a Monday. If they had all the pasta in the jar on Friday, they would get a treat. For Rex, it was pocket money to save up for a video game. Carol said she couldn't believe how upset Rex would get over a tiny piece of pasta coming out of the jar. It was simple but effective.

I started using this type of reward system, and I remember it worked well. It was all about positivity and reinforcement of good behaviour. When Seren would do something right, the dried pasta that had been removed for hitting the dog would go back into the jar.

We continued with this for a few months, and Seren's treat would always be sweeties from the village sweetie shop that we passed on the way home from school. Even though Seren's behaviour was still not great, she was keeping her pasta in the jar on Friday and getting her weekly sweets, so why then would we change this method?

I was brought up in the 70s when parents used quotes like, 'Children should be seen and not heard'; 'If you do that again you will get a mighty one' – (AKA, smack on the bottom with a shoe); 'If I have to tell you one more time, you will be in so much trouble'; 'Do as you're told'. That's what all parents seemed to say to kids, and that type of parenting is still around now; although, there are some swear words in there now too!

If it didn't cause me any harm, maybe Seren did need some punishment – time-out, a little smack on the hand, just a little short, sharp tap so she would know that she had overstepped the line.

I wasn't entirely sold on the pasta in the jar method as I felt that while it was managing Seren's behaviour in one sense, she was still completely out of control and badly behaved. I had to find another way, so I started talking to friends about what they did, and I realised very quickly that all my friends didn't seem to be going through any problems with their children. I then started to feel quite isolated and different, and it began to affect my self-esteem as I was quite convinced that Seren's behaviour was my fault.

'Magic 1,2,3'

By the time Seren was five, her behaviour wasn't getting any better, in fact, it was probably getting worse. When children are three or four years old, you can make excuses for their tantrums, outlandish and unreasonable behaviours. But when they are five, you start to notice that they are different to their peers or siblings. By now, Daisy was only one and she was still as good as gold. Seren was now in Year1, with a new teacher who was very supportive.

I stumbled across 'Magic 1,2,3' on the internet as I was researching 'how to make your child listen and do as they're told', or something like that. I read lots of great reviews about this wondrous style of parenting, so I decided to order the DVD.

When we received the DVD, I couldn't wait to watch it! After getting Seren to bed, which took about an hour, I joined Karl downstairs, poured us a glass of wine, and watched the DVD eagerly. I think it went on for about three hours. We actually fell asleep watching it, but it had done its job and I was confident that the next day was going to be a very different day!

We woke up excited that today was going to change everything. Thomas Phelan, the founder of 'Magic 1,2,3', referred to young children as 'wild animals'. He went on to discuss the fact that there was simply no point trying to explain to a young child what they had done wrong. He said that there was no point in saying, 'Eat your dinner, some kids are starving and would give anything to eat your dinner right now', or 'Why did you draw crayon all over the walls, that made Mummy upset and it will be very expensive to put that right'. He explained that children's brains weren't wired to realise that children in the world were starving so that means they should eat their carrots. To them, the carrots just look disgusting and they don't want to eat them.

It made sense to us, and we couldn't wait to start putting his concept into action. The plan was that if Seren refused to do as she was told, we would simply say very calmly, 'That's one'. Then we would wait ten seconds before saying, 'Seren, that's two'. We would give her three warnings and if Seren didn't carry out the action by the time we counted to three, she would be put in time-out in her bedroom for a minute of each year, which to us meant five minutes.

That following morning, after watching the DVD, Karl brought me my coffee and gave me a kiss and left as he always did at 7.15 am for work. I went over and over everything that I had watched last night. How would I get her in her room? *How would I keep her in her bedroom? What about Daisy, would she be ok? Was I ready for this*? I heard Seren's door creep open, took a deep breath and gave her a big smile as she walked into the bedroom.

The first few seconds whenever Seren came into the bedroom were always beautiful. With her big blue eyes and gorgeous blonde curls, she would give me a big hug and we would exchange good mornings and kisses. That first couple of minutes where magical and I would always be dumbfounded at how quickly the mood could change, sometimes in a matter of minutes. Seren was able to turn the house from calm into utter chaos before it was even light outside.

The morning went pretty well with this new type of parenting. If Seren wasn't doing what she was told, I would go through the numbers as per the DVD. Seren thought it was quite funny when I would calmly say, 'That's one'. She even giggled, saying, 'Mummy, why are you talking in that funny voice?' At first that was worrying, as Seren was apparently used to me shouting and not used to my 'calm voice'! She also asked, 'Why do you keep counting?'

I actually can't remember whether Seren had any time-outs on that first morning, but I do remember that I felt calmer, the house was calmer, and I was more in control as a parent. Seren went to school that day with no problems at all, and even collecting her from school was easier.

Later that night, Seren and I were playing outside in the garden when Daddy arrived home. I went into the house to finish dinner, and Karl stayed outside with Seren while she played. Karl later told me that while they were outside, he had started with the new type of parenting. Seren had then said to him, 'How do you know about that?' She was shocked that Daddy knew all about the counting too. This certainly makes you realise how innocent they are!

We continued using 'Magic 1,2,3', and although Seren's behaviour was still the same, we felt that it was working for us. It gave us some behaviour management; it made us feel like we were somehow managing the bad behaviour. We constantly told friends about our new way of parenting, but most of them insisted that they felt they didn't need it as their children weren't that bad. I always thought they were lying until we had Daisy. We then realised that they must have thought we were slightly mad, as we were always going on about our 'spirited child'.

Not quite a happy family

I liked feeling normal, feeling the same as everyone else. I had felt so different to everyone else for all of my teenage years, so when we had Seren, I had started to feel 'normal'. 'Fake it until you make it', is a phrase that I knew well. Most of my friends thought I was completely together; however, little did they know I was far from it.

One of the things that I have come to discover is that while you can fake it outside the home, it's usually impossible to fake it behind closed doors. *Was Seren becoming a product of me? Were my personality and my behaviour affecting her? Is this the reason that all our friends seem to be getting it right? They had come from normal families; they appear to have normal lives. Was this Seren's downfall, was the truth now becoming apparent through her?*

I have since learnt that very few people talk about what happens behind closed doors. One of the reasons that I have written this book is to show other parents what can go on behind the smiles. Even the happiest people with the brightest lights can be fighting a battle that we know nothing about.

I continued to play out the happiest of families to all my friends and relatives. I had a loving husband and three beautiful children, yet at night, I would cry myself to sleep because I couldn't cope with my eldest child.

Bedtimes were and have always been an absolute nightmare. It would take no time at all to put Daisy and Flynn to bed, but it could take hours to get Seren to bed, and it was exhausting. Screaming fits, gasping for breath, spitting, crying ... why was this so hard? What were we doing wrong?

Karl and I were being given so much conflicting advice from family and friends on how to parent Seren. Their advice would always be very good, but it would never work. Their advice would work on 'less spirited children' but a childlike Seren was a constant battle.

One of the hardest things we have ever had to do, was to realise that Seren wasn't normal! All the 'normal' bad behaviour books and advice was falling on deaf ears, as Seren's behaviour was spiralling out of control.

Chapter Two

Going 'Down Under', in more ways than one

I had wished on so many stars, so many eyelashes, and asked the Universe so many times to make our dream come true. However, as soon as we set foot in Australia, things went from bad to worse. I wasn't sure if instead of my dream coming true, they had got it wrong and given me my worst nightmare.

After a wonderful yet emotional Christmas, on the 13th of January (13 being my lucky number and weirdly my dad's and my late grandma's too), we left the UK shores and started our big journey to Perth, Australia. Flynn was four months old, Daisy was just two and Seren had just turned six.

Why Australia?

We had been planning the move to Australia for years. Karl's brother, Billy, had migrated there twenty years ago, and whenever we would visit, we would feel sad when we landed back on British soil again. We fell madly in love with the people, the beaches, the weather and the vibe, and we had hoped that one day we would get an opportunity to move there. Finally, Karl was given a wonderful job opportunity in Australia, so of course we couldn't let this pass. Happily we packed up all we had and shipped it, and ourselves, across to the other side of the world.

Saying goodbye to the UK

Little did I know how painful it would be to say goodbye to my friends and family, and just how much it would affect our little family. I honestly felt like my heart broke in two when I said goodbye to my dad. I have always been extremely close to him, so to say goodbye was tremendously hard.

We had a pretty close family. I had my step mum, Karen, my dad, and my younger brother, Josh. Sadly, I hadn't seen my birth mother or half brother and sister for a long time, but I would need to write another book to explain those relationships. As I mentioned before, my dad had remarried when I was fifteen. He and Karen conceived Josh, and even though there was a sixteen-year age gap, we have always been really close. I loved this normality (here I go again with the 'normal'), so saying goodbye to them was very difficult.

Karl's mum, his sister and her young family, our aunts and uncles, as well as our cousins also lived in the UK. Sometimes you don't often realise how close you are as a family until you have to say goodbye. But they were all happy for us and could understand why we were making the move.

One of the things that Karl was so excited about was moving closer to his brother. Billy had lived in Perth since he was sixteen. During this time, he and his wife, Lucy, were expecting twins, so it was an exciting time for us to be moving to Australia.

Karl's dad had moved to Australia twenty-years before, and although Karl didn't speak to him that much, he was still thrilled to know that soon he would be able to see his brother and his dad a lot more.

Bound for Australia

Even though it was heartbreaking to leave our family and friends, we were eager to start a new life in Australia. I was fascinated with the country. I also knew that it was a wonderful place to live and raise a family. I was eager to begin this new chapter of our lives. Karl was looking forward to starting his new job and I was looking forward to focusing on the children and setting up a new family home for us.

However, I was a little unsettled by the fact that we didn't have a large circle of family or friends to find support from, and it was this fact that was to become a real problem in the coming months.

When we first arrived in Australia, we lived about forty-five minutes from the centre of Perth. We stayed in a holiday rental for about three months while we searched for somewhere more permanent. Baron wasn't exactly the beautiful green luscious Wales that we were used to. It was stiflingly hot and in the middle of nowhere. In fact, it was so far out of Perth that the freeway stopped.

Schooling

The schooling system in Wales in both the primary and infant years (up to age seven) is very laid-back and incorporated lots of 'learn through play' approaches. In the UK, I remember picking Seren up from school and it was like watching a cannonball shoot out of a cannon. She would be bursting with energy and would not want to come home as she'd had too much fun at school.

I had no control over her and would be forced to stand there trying my hardest to cajole her to come home with me. With a toddler running one way and a hungry screaming baby in my arms, I found it so hard to get Seren to return to me. She would be running, hiding, shouting, climbing and had absolutely no intention of coming back to Mummy.

Karl was so much better with her. He used to let her run wild for about thirty minutes and run off all that energy. For me, pickups were very different. I would worry that Daisy may run off somewhere. Flynn needed his afternoon feed, and I didn't feel that comfortable breastfeeding him among all the other parents (which is silly), so I would just want to rush home.

I wish I could go back to that point, with the realisation that Seren had been cooped up in the school classroom all afternoon and she needed to run and run and run. I wish I could have told myself to just chill out and let her run – just smile, breath, look at the trees and enjoy this beautiful life that I had.

But I didn't, and every day I would try so hard to get Seren to hold my hand, be like all the other children and just walk home.

Family members would tell me how ridiculous it was that I had to wait until she was ready to come. She was naughty. She was defiant, and I was not parenting her correctly. I wish I had realised that Seren needed that release, instead of trying to fit into society and be like everyone else.

Seren was not like everyone else and it would take me another four years to realise this –to understand that she was different and that was ok, different is great!

But back in those days I didn't – Flynn would be screaming, Daisy crying, and I just wanted Seren to 'COME HERE NOW'!

Which new school?

Before leaving the UK, we always knew that Seren probably wouldn't stay in the first Australian school we chose for her. We had spoken to lots of people and we felt that as she was only six, she would be ok with these coming changes. However, I have since learnt that a lot goes on in a six-year-old's head! They have worries, anxieties, fears, and they feel sadness too, just like adults.

Seren went through a lot when we first moved. She also had to say goodbye to her family, her friends, including her best friend who she had known since she was three. I was probably so driven by creating this 'perfect' life for my children in Australia, that I didn't stop to consider how my eldest daughter would be feeling.

After much research, we found ourselves discussing the positives of sending Seren to a Montessori school. This was to be very different from the small village public school in Wales, but we felt it would suit her.

One of the things that all of her teachers would say was that she would get so engrossed in a task or project that they would struggle to get her to leave that task and start something new. As Montessori schools allow children to independently move from task to task, we felt this type of schooling would be perfect for Seren.

Seren also loved to help me outside with the gardening and collecting eggs (we had chickens and a vegetable garden at our home in Wales). Montessori was all about this – growing vegetables, looking after their chickens, beehives and worming farms. Seren enjoyed doing all of this and found it fascinating. So I fully believed that this type of schooling experience would benefit her.

I didn't enjoy school from about the age of thirteen, so I felt if we could give Seren a different type of education, maybe it would help her. We didn't have a diagnosis before we left the UK, but one thing's for sure, we knew at age six that Seren was different from the other children.

The Montessori school

After chatting with friends and family, I started to feel that the Montessori classroom with its endless choice of activities would be perfect for Seren. I felt that as she had the attention span of a gnat, being able to move from task to task whenever she chose would be ideal for her! The Montessori learning approach was very nurturing, very kind, and teachers would observe the children more, instead of just 'teaching' them. There was more interest in nature, in friendships, in the planet. It felt like it would be the answer for Seren and I felt so lucky that there were so many Montessori schools in Perth to choose from.

At the beginning of her new schooling, we would drop her off every morning and she would run in, smiling and happy. Honestly, her resilience astounded me; however, this soon changed. The school, in my opinion, was very strict and so was the teacher. Seren would cry every night and say that the teacher would tell her she was very behind in class. Even though we felt passionate about the Montessori system, we realised very quickly that that particular school wasn't right for Seren, so I started to look at other schools.

I felt so happy when I found another fantastic Montessori school that took Seren immediately. Six weeks later, we moved into our new home and Seren started her new school. Every morning we travelled to school following the road along the sea. We loved the beauty of the ocean, and we all said 'good morning ocean' as we drove by it. We would play Frank Sinatra or the Beach Boys and life felt great. We felt like we were in exactly the right place at the right time. We had found 'home' and it felt wonderful.

After a couple of weeks at the new school, I went to see Seren's teacher for a chat about how she was getting on. Things had been challenging at home, but we were so used to that – it was just 'the norm'. Seren seemed to be more hyperactive and her defiance was getting worse, but whenever I had spoken to teachers in the past, they had always said that things were fine.

Seren's reading hadn't always been the best. She didn't enjoy reading and she was unable to concentrate when I would read to her in bed. One night I had decided to read Black Beauty to her. She had loved the film and a friend bought her the book, thinking she would like to read the story. Daisy was mesmerised by the book and all the wonderful illustrations of the horses, especially the beautiful Black Beauty. Even though we thought it would be Seren's favourite book (at age six she still didn't have one), she left the bed and started to do snow angels or sand angels (as we now lived in Australia) on the floor. But there was no snow or sand, just carpet, so I guess you would call them 'carpet angels'. Whatever they were, they were annoying the hell out of me and made me frustrated!

Why can't she just sit down and read a book like a normal child? Why after six years did she still not have a favourite book, one that she would ask us to read every night? And why, oh why, does she jump on the bed, writhe around, do cartwheels, do handstands, refuse to brush her teeth and protest at going to bed? Every. Single. Night! What is wrong with Seren?

I remember going to meet the teacher and feeling so excited and happy that we had made the right decision with this particular school. I loved the school, loved the teachers, the parents and the other children, and I was convinced that we were giving Seren and the rest of the children a wonderful life.

My happiness soon turned to sadness as I listened intently to Seren's teacher as she explained how Seren was hyperactive, behind in both reading and writing, and she was not making friends. She told me that although the children liked her, they seemed very wary of her, often not understanding her or trusting her, as she was so excitable and 'spirited'. *Here we go with that word 'spirited' again; it's starting to follow us around!*

She told me that Seren often acted like the 'class clown' and the other children would just stare at her in amazement. She told me that Seren was very hyper, very anxious and would move from task to task with no method or understanding of what she was doing. She couldn't decide where to sit during class, where to sit for morning tea, who to sit with, and was usually jumping around disturbing all the other children. The teacher also went to on to say that she had never come across anyone like Seren before. Although the children seemed wary of her, she was very popular and a born leader, often directing the children on how to do their work (even though Seren wasn't sure what she was supposed to be doing).

The teacher felt very strongly though that, with the right guidance and nurturing, Seren would do very well at the school. I felt very lucky to have finally found someone who had 'seen' what we had seen in Seren. And I thought that maybe together we could all help Seren.

I agreed with everything the teacher told me as it pretty much summed up our little six-year-old daughter. Also, by now, my trusted 'Magic 1,2,3' wasn't working anymore, and Seren was definitely too big for the naughty step now! We had tried everything – every reward system, every type of parenting – all had failed and I now found myself shouting and screaming at her over everything and anything. I had also smacked her a couple of times, something I was not proud of. However, when you have nothing else to try, you start to believe that maybe the old-fashioned way of parenting was the answer.

Is it ADHD?

I remember mentioning to family members that maybe Seren could be suffering from ADHD. We all felt that because Seren could focus on her favourite TV program or immerse herself in art and crafts for extended periods of time, she couldn't possibly have ADHD. At the time we knew very little about it, but we assumed that children with ADHD couldn't focus on anything.

I have since learnt that what Seren had was actually called 'hyper-focus'. If an ADHD child is interested in something, they can become so focused on what they are doing that it is almost impossible to get them to move onto something else.

Seren had no interest in books, reading or writing, but she loved to draw. She loved numbers and she would move from project to project like a mad scientist – play with the dolls, play with the kitchen, play with the dog, make a den, run outside, run back in, play with a jigsaw, watch TV. Seren would move from one thing to another with no structure or rhyme or reason.

I recall one day when Seren was about eighteen months old. I had been silently sitting on the floor in her bedroom watching her in amazement. She was running around her room; she would climb in the cot, then climb out, climb on the chair, then climb down, hide in the wardrobe, then pop back out again. I called Karl and he joined me on the carpet, just watching her in bewilderment. It was like she'd been given an adrenalin shot and she continued making this haphazard pattern for about fifteen minutes, not even noticing us sitting there watching her. Even 'spirited' didn't explain her behaviour – she was chaotic and hyper at such a young age.

Friends to talk to

I was so excited when one of the mums at the new school asked me to go for coffee. We had met in the school car park after I asked her about her baby carrier. We realised that we had children of similar ages and started to regularly chat about kids, life and school, and then one day, Frankie asked me if I would like to go for coffee.

It's funny how friendships start. In the UK, I had known all my friends since I was fifteen, some even younger, and we had built strong, trusting relationships over that time. My best friends in the UK knew every single thing about me, but this new territory was very different – it felt like dating again! I had been very spoilt in the UK, and I didn't ever really try to make new friends while I lived there. However, with a new life in a new country, I had to start making new friends, otherwise I was going to feel completely alone and isolated forever.

Karl looked after Daisy and Flynn, and I skipped off to meet Frankie. We met in a coffee shop and as we sat drinking coffee and eating cake, we talked about life, dreams, husbands, and kids. It became apparent that we had more in common than I first thought. I spoke to Frankie about Seren's behaviour and even though I barely knew her, I found myself telling her my darkest secrets, my deepest feelings and fears about my daughter.

I had no-one else to talk to, and although I spoke to my parents and my best friend, they were 9,000 miles away. And even after spending hours on the phone with them, I have come to learn that there is nothing better than real human interaction. There were also times when I couldn't confide in them about how hard things were as I didn't want to worry them. I also felt awful about complaining about things when we had this amazing new life in Australia.

I honestly believe this is why so many people are struggling in today's society. My grandma used to tell me stories of how she would talk over the fence with her neighbours and friends, and how that all stopped when the houses were knocked down, and high-rise flats were built after the war. My grandma, along with many others, felt that it changed communities and society overnight – friends couldn't talk over the fence like they used to and people were more isolated.

I guess life has become like that even more now; it's so over-complicated. There is no-one to talk to over the fence anymore and, even if you did, it could be all over social media in a heartbeat! Even worse, there would be video evidence as someone would have recorded it and put it up on a social media site. And then what would that do to our image? Everyone is trying to portray through social media that everything in life is perfect; however, we all know it's far from it.

Frankie has since become one of my dearest friends and has been there for me when I was at my lowest. I never did actually tell her when I was at my lowest, I tried so hard to keep that covered, but our weekly doggy and toddler walks after school drop-offs were a great sense of relief as we talked and walked for hours.

Should we see someone?

It was actually Frankie who suggested that I take Seren to see a specialist. She knew of a great psychologist who had diagnosed a friend's child with anxiety and she thought that maybe it was worth taking Seren to be assessed. I had never heard of anxiety in children before, but I have since realised that, unfortunately, it's a disorder of our times. Sadly, more and more children are being diagnosed with this disorder as they are struggling to cope in this ever-changing, fast-paced world.

Seren is full-on and hyperactive, but anxious? I am pretty sure that she isn't anxious – could a six-year-old even have 'anxiety'? Wasn't anxiety just something that happened to adults? We had lots to be concerned about – relationships, kids, debt, work, illness, addiction, cancer, terrorists! It's never-ending and one of the reasons why I rarely watch TV or read the papers. I want to stay in my 'Susy bubble', as it's much safer there!

But how can a loved, wanted, nurtured child be anxious? What on earth would a six-year-old child need to be anxious about? Choosing their cereal? What to watch on TV? Whether to read The Secret Seven *or* James and the Giant Peach *– I mean, come on?*

But how wrong and naive I was!

Frankie told me about a child psychologist who had a keen interest in play therapy – children would play games, create arts and craft with her and not be aware that they were being assessed. She had personally used this therapist and found her very honest and helpful, so she sent me her number.

I called the psychologist the very next day and made an appointment to see her a week or so later. At the same time, I booked in to see our GP and explained to him all about Seren, her defiance, her hyperactivity, and how we were struggling to cope. He told me that he would make an appointment for us to see a pediatrician as well, but the waiting lists were long. He made a couple of phone calls and each pediatrician's office told him that they had a twelve-month waiting list.

This was the first indication that behind the long stretches of white sand, the sparkling turquoise waters and the everlasting sunshine, lay a dark secret; however, even at that moment, nothing could have prepared me for what lay ahead for us – what lay ahead for Seren.

I later found out that many of the child psychiatrists and psychologists had closed their books, as they simply couldn't handle any more patients. *How can they have so many children on their books? What is wrong with all the kids and why did they all need to see professionals?*

After making some more phone calls, our GP finally found a pediatrician who only had a three-month waiting list. The GP wrote a letter to the pediatrician and advised me that he would be in contact shortly with a date, but we would be looking at some time in August.

I felt apprehensive, but I also felt like I had made the right decision as we had struggled with Seren for six years. We had no idea how to parent her, and our family and closest friends in the UK also didn't know how to handle her.

We had also noticed that Seren often couldn't look us in the eye, she found it hard to stay focused when having a conversation and her eyes would wander constantly. Although I didn't feel that she did this to me a lot, Karl felt that he didn't have a loving relationship with Seren and it upset him. Most nights Karl would put Seren to bed, and then either Karl or myself would put Daisy to bed. He would fight with Seren every night – she would be screaming, he would be frustrated – it was a daily battle. Putting to bed a six-month-old baby and a two-year-old toddler could be done and dusted in no time, but putting our six year old to bed could take an hour or longer, and we would be emotionally exhausted by the end of it. We should have been masters at doing it, as Seren had been like that ever since we took her out of the cot when she was two, but we weren't masters and it was getting harder and harder.

Maybe Seren did need to see a professional? Maybe this was the answer? Maybe some parents struggle to know what to do, and a professional can help? It's not like children come with a book of instructions; wouldn't that be amazing!

First, you birth the baby and then a 'guide to parenting them' popped out with handy tips for each year of their life. What a fabulous idea, if only there was an app for that!

Unfortunately, that wasn't the case. I'd read so many books, tried so many parenting methods and watched so many parenting programs that my head was in a spin.

It's interesting to point out here that, because Seren had always been difficult, even as a toddler we had always gone down the 'naughty step' route. We hadn't tried the 'calm, ignore the bad, praise the good' type parenting, so I will never know if this would have made a difference. I have come to learn that this would have been a much better way of parenting Seren – it's a shame we don't have time machines.

However, I have learnt that if a child is 'labelled' hyperactive, strong-willed, spirited, naughty, defiant, or has ADHD, ASD, ODD – whatever you want to call it – punishment was not the answer!

We didn't want Seren labelled and we knew that would happen if we took her to a specialist. But we felt we had no other choice; we were out of our depth and something needed to change.

First trip to the psychologist

Our appointment to see the child psychologist came along, so with Daisy and Flynn asleep in the buggy (thank you, Lord, for these simple, wondrous moments), we sat with the psychologist for an hour giving her an overview of Seren, her behaviour, our family life, our parenting and our relationship.

I remember Karl and me being quite emotional as we talked about our non-existent relationship with our six-year-old and how it was impacting so negatively on our family dynamic. Our meeting was very thorough, and many private and personal questions were asked, which we were happy to answer honestly and truthfully.

I felt guilty, overwhelmed and was starting to feel that some of these problems were solely my fault. I felt like the blame was being pointed towards me more than Karl. He talked about my anger and how he felt the situation seemed to bother me more than it bothered him.

I spoke about growing up, my mother's struggles with alcohol addiction, and my parent's constant arguing and fighting as a child. Karl explained how his dad had left when he was eleven years old, and how his mum had raised him, his brother and sister, with love and nurturing – he hadn't come from a family where aggression prevailed. However, Karl also came from a broken marriage – it's one of the things that bound us together sixteen years ago. When we first met, when I was just twenty-three, we told each other how it felt when our parents divorced and the impact that it had on us as children. We had similar paths in a way: Karl hadn't had much of a relationship with his father after he moved to Australia, and I hadn't had a relationship with my mum since I was a teenager.

We had very similar views on parenting, life, hopes and dreams, yet in this meeting I was starting to feel like some of the problems we were facing were my fault, as I was the one with a quick temper. I was the one who could get upset with Seren and quickly lose control of the situation.

The psychologist suggested seeing Seren weekly for ten weeks. She would assess her through play and then meet with us again to discuss the findings, with a plan of action.

We had feelings of relief and happiness, and although we were worried what the outcome may be, we felt at ease that we were finally doing something about it. We were finally sharing our story with a professional and felt confident that they would know what was wrong with Seren – surely they would know how to fix our family!

Regular trips

Every Thursday I would collect Seren from school after lunch and we would head to see the psychologist. Seren loved going, as she would get one-on-one time with the therapist. I used to feel incredibly guilty that I wasn't able to spend more time with Seren one-on-one. I felt that maybe things would be different if I did. However, as anyone with a challenging child knows, time together can be so hard that you often find yourself wishing the time away!

Waiting ten weeks

Ten weeks seemed to go by pretty quickly, although it got harder and harder to cope with Seren's on-going behaviour. I would lose her virtually every time we would go out – the beach, especially, became a never-ending nightmare.

I remember being at the beach once with a friend when I suddenly realised I had lost Seren. Daisy was right next to me playing with a bucket and spade, and Flynn was asleep, but where was Seren? Although Seren could swim well for her age, I started to look frantically ahead into the ocean, fearing that she has been abducted or drowned! I ran, screaming up and down the beach, trying desperately to find her. My mind raced and people around me started to help look for her. I seemed to have no systematic way of looking for her and didn't know where to start first. I checked the toilets, the park, the cafe, all the while thinking, *Oh my god where is she?* I ran along the beach back and forth, and then in the distance I noticed Seren fishing on some rocks with a little girl and her dad. *Fishing? Why on earth is she fishing and why didn't she ask me or tell me?* I screamed at her and she came running. I yelled across the beach at her, and the dad was looking at me like I had gone completely and utterly mad.

There have been moments when I have lost sight of Daisy at the park, but it was only for a few seconds and then she'd reappear out from the slide or I would notice her little foot peeping out from the climbing frame. But Seren, I have lost Seren countless times for minutes, and those minutes have seemed like a lifetime. I was so over it and I knew that we were making the right decision by seeing a specialist. *How many times can you lose your child?* It was getting out of hand.

The verdict

Ten weeks later, the day arrived when Karl and I would meet with the psychologist. I remember making an effort with my clothes that day, and instead of wearing my usual 'Mummy got out of bed and threw anything on' style, I made a real effort, dressing in smart trousers, a blouse and brogues. *Why did I do that? Did it mean that I was somehow a better mother if I wore smart clothes?* I styled my hair, put on some makeup, and Karl and I left to see the psychologist.

When we arrived, Daisy and Flynn were peacefully asleep in the double buggy (thank you lunchtime sleeps). At least I could do something right! I had two peacefully sleeping little bunnies, so I wasn't that much of a failure.

What's the verdict going to be? Is it all just down to bad parenting? Is Seren autistic? She isn't very good at eye contact; she doesn't have any empathy and gets lost in her own world? Is it this?

Feelings of regret and guilt over giving her childhood vaccinations now started to enter my mind, my thoughts raced and whirled around in my head like a twister and I was unable to think of anything else as we entered the psychologist's office.

And then the moment of truth ...

I will never forget the sinking words of the psychologist: 'Your daughter has Attention Deficit Hyperactivity Disorder (ADHD) and she is at the extreme end. She also has anxiety. My advice is that you medicate her with Ritalin.'

What? No? Really? How? Why? What did I do wrong?

I suddenly felt myself fall into a blind panic, as all I'd ever heard about ADHD was that it was down to bad parenting, poor diet, and a lack of discipline. We had only just moved to Australia. I had dreamt of long hot summers, the children playing outside until sunset, and endless days swimming in the ocean. Yet, here I was three months into our journey with my world crashing around me.

I was so upset that I started to cry. When I glanced over at Karl, he had tears in his eyes too – it was crushing.

What's more, during this past month, Seren was probably the worst she had ever been. She was hyperactive, defiant and out of control. She wasn't able to obey a simple instruction. She was mean to her brother and sister. She would run away, scream, throw things and slam doors. She would tell me she hated me. She would scream at me to leave her alone, yelling, 'I'm not part of this family'. Many times she would yell at me, 'Shut up you fat, old woman' – that one particularly hurt, as I was approaching forty!

I may be able to joke about this now, but at the time it was crushing. She was still only six years old. I thought we would have to wait until her teens before this kind of verbal abuse started! She would also regularly scream and hit out at Karl. There were times when it would drive him to tears as his beautiful daughter attacked him physically and verbally. Even writing this now brings tears to my eyes.

Diary entries after Seren was diagnosed with ADHD

8 May

Seren was defiant this morning. She wouldn't listen to anything I said, and weirdly she started to strip Flynn's bedclothes off his bed instead of getting ready for school. Even though I asked her to get dressed, she put on a DVD. She takes so long to do things – get dressed, make her bed, put on her shoes. Everything is a battle. She wouldn't wear her coat, even though it was raining. She screamed that she would never wear it. I tried to force it on, but she then ran and hid. She said she hates me, ran off throwing her coat on the floor outside.

15 May

Seren was fantastic today. My mood was terrible, but she was better! She asked for her jobs and we put the list of them up on the fridge. She seemed so much better today. I am not giving her apple juice or chocolate spread again now after yesterday. Trying to watch what she eats as I know there is a link. Great day with Seren!

19 May

Seren had been great all weekend and then this morning was terrible. She did go to Scitech yesterday, was it this? Was it too much stimulation? I found her watching the iPad too. Was it that? She couldn't read her list of things to do in the morning. She wouldn't eat her breakfast? She wouldn't wear her clothes or put on her sunscreen. She was aggressive, rude, obnoxious! She went out of the house this morning screaming, 'Get away from me, I hate you'. Bad day. :-(

26 May

Screaming uncontrollably, hitting out, hysterical, kicking, it got so bad today that I smacked her on her hand. I was so upset afterwards as this isn't the type of mum I want to be. I feel like we have tried everything, I just don't know what to do. I honestly can't cope anymore. It is impossible to function as a family with this behaviour. I am at my wit's end. I am so upset. I feel so lonely and don't know what to do. Help. :-(

No-one knew

It's still hard to read these honest diary entries. This was my 'real life' but no-one knew what we were going through at the time, how difficult our life really was.

I think we are all guilty of 'pretending' so well these days. Everyone is trying to portray this amazing, happy life. We try and show the world that we are in control of our lives – that our kids are well behaved, our house is clean and tidy, and our relationships are perfect. And sometimes we fall off the 'perfect' wagon and our true feelings come out through social media. People vent how they feel about their kids, their partners, their jobs, or the government, but then the next day they go back to their perfect children, their perfect lives and so it continues. Social media has a lot to answer for! Yes, there is a place for it – we can connect with like-minded people all over the world, we can find out any piece of information at the touch of a button; however, just like personalities, it has a dark side.

I was going through one of the scariest, darkest times in my life and yet if I look back on my Facebook pictures, my life seemed like a dream! Life isn't perfect and deep down we all know that, yet we still succumb to this nonsense. *What is it all about?* We are busy posting pictures of our perfect life, with our perfect kids, our tidy, clean house and our perfect 'beach wave' hair, because we can't tell people, 'You know what, my life is hell right now. My eldest daughter is seeing a psychologist and I don't know how to cope with her behaviour!'

Was it because we were in Australia?

When we moved to Australia, Seren's behaviour started to get worse, much worse.

At this point, we didn't know anyone with ADHD; it was something that had never crossed our paths. We left the UK when most of our friends' children were six or younger. *Perhaps as the children get older, they might be diagnosed? Maybe they won't? Maybe it's because people don't discuss this, it's a taboo after all. Or maybe it's because none of my friends in the UK have problems with their kids? Maybe it's because we moved to Australia where it seems more commonplace?*

It's so interesting, though, as I know so many people in Australia who's children have been diagnosed with something. It seems here in Australia there is a label for just about anything to do with childhood – too much sneezing, yep there's a label; too much giggling, yep another label; singing in the shower, definitely a label!

I know I am being silly, but I do wonder what I would have been labelled with had I been born twenty years later. Forgetful, clumsy, excitable, emotional – I probably would have accumulated as many as three or four labels to my name! It's not the letters after your name that are important now – the new buzz is 'labels'. Susy O'Hare ADHD, ODD, dyspraxia, dyslexia ... is the world a better place now we all have these labels, or is it a world gone mad?

I am sure it would have occurred in any country that we lived in, as ADHD rates seem to be increasing all over the world.

So what does it all mean?

ADHD is now a word that is associated with raising children. Every parent knows of a child who has ADHD, or their own child has this disorder. The name is whispered in the school corridors and mothers chat anonymously to each other on internet forums. But due to the stigma, no-one talks about it openly. However, it's there, and ADHD is growing in numbers globally, like a silent cancer.

At the time of Seren's diagnosis, I had every Tom, Dick and Harry telling me that ADHD was an illness, a disorder, a disability. So, I decided to look into it further myself. I was determined to learn all I could about this 'illness' and look into other ways, rather than medication, to help her. I had to know that I had looked at all options first; however, in a medical world that only really supports drugs, it was so hard to find out what the options were.

One of the most important things I learnt was that 'change' had an adverse affect on ADHD kids. When we moved, we had essentially taken Seren away from everyone she knew – her friends, her family, her home and her school. Everyone tells us that kids are resilient and they just get on with it, and we think that kids are bombproof. We believe that we can say anything to them and they will be alright, but you know what, they are just the same as adults – just a smaller version.

They get scared. They get worried, anxious and frightened, yet children don't understand their feelings so they express them through emotions and anger. The more we pushed Seren away, the worse her behaviour became, but it would take a long time for us to realise this.

It's so strange when you have a child with a 'mental illness'. Having gone through the journey, I personally don't fully believe that ADHD is a mental illness, but I do know that it can carry with it feelings of anxiety and depression. For me, the depression and anxiety side of ADHD is a mental illness, but I believe that ADHD is just how you are made up. I hope that, over time, this 'taboo' is set free, instead of allowing parents to think that something is wrong with their child.

Until I went through this journey with Seren, I would never have imagined that a six-year-old child could have anxiety or depression. What I know now is that mental illness can happen to anyone at any time, and the way in which we generally handle mental illness is so wrong.

Medicate or not?

There is still a huge stigma surrounding mental illness, but the use of antidepressants and medication is becoming normalised, especially in children, which I don't believe is the answer either. Medication helps a lot of children and a lot of families, and I am not knocking this, but were we really meant to evolve to only be able to succeed in life through popping pills? *What has gone wrong? What has happened to us as a race? Is this the way it is supposed to be?* I wonder what the animal kingdom must think of us – if only they could talk!

Medication can fix one thing, but then it brings along a host of side effects, which then also need 'fixing'. So then more drugs are needed, and the cycle continues until you are not sure what the medicine is helping and what it's causing.

I say this from experience. Medication helped Seren in many ways, but it also produced scary side effects, many that I didn't realise until after she stopped taking medication. For a long time I thought it was just us; I figured it was just Seren who was having side effects. The drugs seemed to work for other families; they all appeared to be fine. Then I came to realise that this wasn't the case at all, and what happened to Seren was just the tip of the iceberg, as it was also happening to many others around the world.

When we asked the psychologist about other methods for ADHD, she only recommended medication. She said it was the best-proven type of treatment for ADHD and she also suggested seeing Seren weekly to help her with her anxiety. Immediately, I questioned whether this was the right choice for our child.

At age six, let's just medicate her and make everything go away! It will make it all better, like giving a child ice-cream when they have a sore throat; it will make her smile, and feel happier, it will make everything alright again. But is this the answer? Medicate my young child?

I am not against medication; I understand it has a place, and for countless families it is helping them live a somewhat normal life, but surely there had to be another more natural approach?

No-one knows what they're doing

I felt like I couldn't just accept the medication before I had tried every other type of help, but I very quickly learnt that, just like parenting, no-one else knows what they are doing! This is why there are so many different ways to birth a child, raise a child, and parent a child.

Is everyone just flying by the seat of their pants?

One of the best quotes I have read was by the comedian and actor Ricky Gervais, when he said, 'The best advice I've ever received is, "No-one else knows what they are doing either."'

It's important for me to hold this quote in my mind and to remember that it is true in so many ways. The medicating of children has become as routine as buying them a lollipop at the local shop, but it's simply not advertised like that. You don't see kids walking around sucking on their medication lollies, so no-one knows it's going on. However, when you are in it, you realise that it's everywhere and it's getting more normalised with prescriptions rates for children soaring year on year!

More questions should have been asked

I do personally believe in ADHD; it has been proven with brain scans in ADHD children. The psychologist who saw Seren explained to us that these children have lower dopamine levels, which can then cause hyperactivity, impulsivity and a reduction in executive functioning (which is decision-making and thinking of secondary consequences, i.e. not running across the road when a lorry is coming – which Seren often did.)

It has also been proven through brain scans that giving a child stimulant medication increases the dopamine levels and helps the neurotransmitters to work efficiently, which in turn decreases the levels of hyperactivity and impulsivity (i.e. not running across the road when a lorry is coming).

However, unfortunately, children aren't being given brain scans and professionals are just assessing their behaviour, which can often mean that due to other external factors, children are wrongly diagnosed and medicated unnecessarily. This then can lead to more problems and risky, adverse side effects.

When I was pregnant with Flynn, like all pregnant women, I would have my blood pressure checked during my check-ups with the midwife.

One particular day the midwife said that my blood pressure seemed quite high. She said that this could sometimes happen when women were a little nervous, or worried, so she did some other checks and then checked my blood pressure again at the end. After we had chatted and spent some time together, my blood pressure reading was lower, as she predicated. When people go for an operation, it can often be the case that they have more adrenaline running around their body so their blood pressure rating would be higher because they are nervous. The surgeon will take all this into consideration; he/she won't write out a prescription for diuretics, he/she will understand that it is probably due to 'adrenalin'.

What if this happened to Seren every time she saw the psychologist? She had just finished lunch, was it something that she had eaten? Was it something that I had given her to drink? What if I had just given her a can of soft drink and she was high from the sugar rush?

There are so many variables that could have affected her behaviour, so why weren't more questions asked?

Where are the guidelines and why didn't anyone ever talk about the fact that we had just moved countries and that this could be affecting Seren? Or what about the fact that she had changed schools and was missing her friends and family, or she could just be suffering from anxiety that can often manifest itself as 'ADHD'. These were just some of the most pressing questions I had, and so therefore I had to keep researching.

What I did find out was that, in Australia, at least one child in every three is wrongly diagnosed with Attention Deficit Hyperactivity Disorder (ADHD), according to a study led by a leading psychiatrist Dr Jon Jureidini. Dr Jureidini is among a group of concerned doctors who warned the Federal Government's ADHD panel about the alarming surge of ADHD misdiagnosis in Australia, urging the board to revise the current diagnostic guidelines and criteria for ADHD.[2]

Diagnosis instead of Ritalin?

The psychologist recommended that we see a pediatrician as she couldn't give us a prescription for Ritalin, but they could. We explained that we didn't want to medicate Seren, and I insisted that I would find another way. The psychologist went on to explain that it was our choice, but she felt very strongly that we should medicate Seren.

I find it fascinating that, although medication seems to be the choice in Australia, the US, and other countries, some countries like the UK and France aren't so quick to hand out a diagnosis and medication. French child psychiatrists view ADHD as a medical condition that has psychosocial and situational causes. Instead of treating children's focusing and behavioural problems with drugs, French doctors prefer to look for the underlying issue that is causing the child distress. And in doing this, they don't look for problems in the child's brain, but rather the problems in the child's social context. They then choose to treat the underlying social context problem with psychotherapy or family counselling.[3]

At the time of doing all my initial research on ADHD, in 2015, 11% of children in the US had ADHD[4], but this rate is growing year on year. Also, in Australia, 11% of children had ADHD[5], yet in France is it less than 5%[3], with the UK having similar lower numbers[6].

How can double the number of children have ADHD in some countries? Is there something wrong with our medical system or is there something wrong with our children?

From my research, I have learnt that in Australia and the US they use medication as a first response to manage ADHD, whereas in the UK, France and countries such as Denmark, medication is a second response. I wonder how differently our ADHD rates would look if we adopted their method?

What about childbirth?

I'd just like to elaborate on my thoughts about childbirth, initially discussed earlier. Women are the same all over the world. Our bodies don't work differently because we are born in France or Australia. The difference, however, is the medical world. In Australia, we have private medical hospitals, which basically means that the difference is *money.*

I truly believe that our births and our children have become part of a multi-billion dollar industry. Private hospitals in Australia have higher caesarian section rates than public hospitals. In 2011, 43% of women in private hospitals had birth by caesarian section compared with 30% in public hospitals. Around 31% of women in Australia will opt to have their babies in private hospitals, while in the UK only 1% of women will have their babies in a private hospital.[7, 8, 9]

Statistics all around the world show that women are more likely to have a caesarian section if they have their baby in a private hospital, rather than a public hospital. In fact, the difference can be around 20%.[9] Australia has the same percentages as the US for caesarian sections – 32%, and we have the same numbers as the US for ADHD in children, but both numbers are growing year on year.[9]

I understand that there is a need for caesarean births, many of my friends have had caesareans. However, in the birthing world, there are so many experts who feel that we need to ensure that the next generation – all around the world – is born in the best place and in the best way for them. Are we normalising the labelling and medicating of children, just as we are normalising caesarian sections? Our psychologist felt that medication, along with weekly sessions with Seren, would help manage the ADHD. However, I felt that more needed to be done over a longer period before handing out such a life-changing diagnosis.

Particularly when this diagnosis came with a prescription for stimulant medication that comes with side effects. I just couldn't understand when it had become so commonplace to medicate children in the first instance, without looking into other factors.

The psychologist's advice

It was now July, and as suggested I took Seren every Thursday to meet with the psychologist. I would drop Seren off and take Daisy and Flynn to the park across the road. Seren would always come out with sweets, which were a cute idea, but they would send Seren into a hyperactive spin in the car every week!

For a long time, I didn't notice the unbelievable changes that happened to Seren when she had sugar. It still amazes me that sugar is allowed in schools when these children are so sensitive to it. As parents, we all know how children can get a 'sugar rush', and then the 'sugar crash' afterwards. We often make a joke of it! However, what I have realised is that for most ADHD children, it can have a huge effect on their behaviour. This isn't always the case, however, as one of my good friends who has a daughter with ADHD doesn't ever notice a change in her behaviour after sugar. But for Seren, the change is instant – think, 'jumping up and down on all the furniture and running around the house like a Tasmanian devil' type changes!

The psychologist suggested meeting with Karl and me after we had met with the paediatrician in the next few weeks. And so, life continued being crazy and full-on, and yet I didn't tell anyone (well, hardly anyone) that our little girl was diagnosed with this 'illness' and that we were desperately trying to deal with this diagnosis. I couldn't help but feel like it was my fault, that it was something that I had done wrong. I was a bad mother. I was a failure.

So we organised to go to the pediatrician. I think we were desperate to get another diagnosis from the pediatrician – surely he would know what was wrong. He was an expert; we would be in good hands.

Chapter Three

Aladdin's cave

When you go to a doctor and the waiting room is like the best toyshop in town, you smile because you feel you are in good hands – this doctor surely understands children. How strange it can seem to leave the office just minutes later with a prescription for medicated speed.

The big day finally arrived when Seren would see the pediatrician and be assessed. It was a sunny day in August, and Seren wanted to wear a pretty dress that day. She didn't really understand where we were going. We always just said we were seeing someone who might be able to help her with her behaviour. I never stopped to think how that might have made her feel, or what it did to her confidence or her self-esteem. Maybe this was the reason that Seren had the biggest tantrum in the car before we even arrived. She was screaming at me, I was screaming at her, and Karl was trying to calm the situation down.

As I have touched on previously, one of the major things that I have realised through this whole process is that Seren can't handle change and neither can I, so that makes us like two peas in a pod. But we're definitely not green, round, shiny, happy peas sitting next to each other. We are more like angry, screaming peas, bursting out of their pods and upsetting all the other little green peas in their wake! This pretty much summed up my relationship with Seren (although I should have known better, as I was the adult). So after having a screaming match, we calmed down, found our smiles and walked into the pediatrician's office.

Will he do some tests? Brain scans? Talk to Seren at length, test her IQ? What's going to happen? How will he assess her? How will he know?

Let's see what the pediatrician says

We were scared and worried about the diagnosis, but we were also relieved that this day was finally here. The psychologist had diagnosed Seren with ADHD, but what if she was wrong? What if it wasn't ADHD at all? However, I think my gut told me that the diagnosis would be the same. Even though we were worried about seeing the pediatrician, we were happy to finally be seeing an expert, someone who would know what to do. Maybe this was the person who could save Seren – who could save our family.

Walking into the reception was like walking into 'Aladdin's cave', and immediately we felt like we were at the right place. This man surely understood children, as there were toys everywhere! It was certainly a sight for sore eyes for any parent who has a hyperactive child and was dreading the 'waiting' in the waiting room!

We had been waiting for about ten minutes when the pediatrician ushered us all into his room. The Aladdin's cave now turned into a very poky room. The room was so small that only Seren, the pediatrician and myself could fit in there. Karl had to wait outside. There was a bed, weighing scales and two chairs. *How am I supposed to keep Seren in this room for an hour?* We decided that it would be a good idea for Seren to stay with Karl, and that I would answer all the questions with the pediatrician.

I would have to say that he only spent a few minutes with Seren: once briefly chatting to her when she first entered the room, then weighing her and listening to her heartbeat. When the pediatrician listened to Seren's heart, he said that she had a heart murmur. He felt that this wasn't a cause for concern but he was just noting it (I always wondered whether a child with a heart murmur should be given stimulant medication).

He then went on to ask me, what seemed like, hundreds of questions about Seren's behaviour; however, they were all closed questions with me only answering 'yes' to most of them. I felt like I was being led down the garden path and at the bottom was a sign saying, 'Your child has ADHD'.

The meeting went on for about forty-five minutes, and during this time, he had only spoken to Seren for all of two minutes. Two minutes spent talking to a child, the person being assessed, and then just like that – 'Your child has

ADHD'. He also had the report from the psychologist but he clearly stated at the beginning of our meeting that he wouldn't make a diagnosis based on what the psychologist had said, as he would make the final decision. And just as my gut had told me, his decision was that Seren had ADHD and he recommended medicating her immediately with Ritalin.

I asked about fish oils, diet, parenting, and if these could help children with ADHD instead of medication. I was told that the medication usually sorted the problem out and nothing else was needed.

Nothing else is needed, just medication. Is that really advice we are giving now to frantic, desperate parents? That's all you get from these professionals who have studied for eleven plus years after high school!

He didn't seem to care about Seren's diet, our parenting methods, or even seem bothered about checking her blood to see if there was anything wrong with her. It just seemed so crazy, that you could meet a child for only a few minutes, weigh them, listen to their heartbeat and then send them off with a prescription for medication.

We left the pediatrician's office that day with a prescription for Ritalin LA. The pediatrician told me that, apparently under the Australian medical guidelines, pediatricians are supposed to start with Ritalin SA, which only last four hours, before going to Ritalin LA, which lasts for 10–12 hours. As we weren't receiving Medicare at the time, we were paying for our prescriptions so we fell into a loophole, and therefore Seren could be prescribed Ritalin LA.

It just doesn't seem right

Desperate to find answers, and support, I immediately investigated various support groups to join. I spent hours searching on Google and ADHD Facebook groups, but there was so much conflicting advice, I didn't know which way to turn.

And what were we to do when all the experts were telling us to medicate our child? What if I had been feeding my daughter a fast food diet, loading her up with sweets and letting her watch TV and play video games all day and night, surely then this could have made the problem worse.

But there were no questions like this asked. Medication was the first, and only, response.

Lifestyle?

Before moving to Australia, I watched back-to-back episodes of *Wanted Down Under*, and I desperately wished that we could move there. I loved the place, and when it was time to make the move, I couldn't wait to start a new life here.

But when we were finally settled in our new home, I couldn't help but question the fact that we have access to this glorious lifestyle – the sunshine, the outdoors, the beautiful landscape, the rivers, the ocean – so how then are so many children being diagnosed with ADHD? *What was wrong with our children?*

Home births?

Now here's the thing that I find odd. I had natural, home births for Daisy and Flynn, and used no drugs. Flynn didn't even have the vitamin K injection, as he had the cream. I breastfed all three children. I bought organic meat, fruit and vegetables, used chemical-free products on my kids, and in the UK we lived in the country and raised chickens. Yet here I was, six months after we moved, standing in the chemist waiting for a Ritalin prescription.

Why am I doing it? Why am I buying into this madness? Why have I chosen to medicate my child with stimulant medication at age six? Why?

Because ... I believed the psychologist and I believed the pediatrician, but mainly because I was completely and utterly unable to cope with my six-year-old's behaviour. It was so bad and out of control, medication seemed like the only answer!

I was determined to find a natural way to help Seren with her ADHD, but I found it was like trying to find a needle in a haystack. We decided that we would do as was suggested and give her the medication. This would hopefully manage her behaviour and give us all some breathing space whilst I researched and looked into all the other natural methods to manage her ADHD. We felt that when we had found another way, we could stop the medication.

Everyone felt Seren had ADHD, and everyone felt that medication would be better for Seren. But was it better for Seren or was it just better for us?

We were so out of our depth with it – how can you not control your six-year-old? Medication would be quick, it would be instant and it would fix everything – or so we were told.

Food?

Another thing that upsets me is the amount of additives that are added to food. Do you know that most of the very foods that we feed our children contain additives that can cause behavioural problems? And this is usually the case for the food that looks nutritious. For example, rice crackers – the packaging looks very healthy and 'kid friendly' and yet when I researched the ingredients, they were laden with mind-altering additives.

I mean, who in their right mind would put that in food for children? Coupled with the fact that Australia is using chemicals and pesticides that were banned in Canada, and the US, in the 1970s. *How on earth are children supposed to consume all of this, and be ok?* Chemicals in foods, chemicals in shampoos, body wash, toothpaste, sunscreen, things that we use on our children, are destroying our endocrine systems. Autism, cancer, ADHD, are all on the rise, and many experts believe that a lot of these increases are due to the environment that children are being raised in. They even tell us that chemicals are in the water that we are drinking.[10] It is very scary and daunting when you are a parent.

I have learnt all of this throughout the journey, but I didn't know any of this when I was standing in the chemist waiting for the Ritalin prescription. I knew about the Ritalin phenomenon, but I was stressed, so over it, so fed up, that I was prepared to just listen to the experts and do as I was told.

Did I feel embarrassed? A failure? A bad mum for doing it? Of course, I did.

I certainly wasn't going to put it as my Facebook status update – 'Seren got diagnosed with ADHD today and I have just picked up the prescription for Ritalin ... Woo hoo what a great day'! No, I didn't do any of that. I felt sick, anxious, sad and helpless. I was in complete panic mode, stressed beyond myself, confused and frightened for the wellness of my child, as her behaviour was getting more and more difficult to handle.

And my dreams of the perfect family were now tumbling around me. I felt that I had no other option. We had seen two experts and both of them had assured us that Seren had ADHD and the best thing would be to medicate her with Ritalin.

I was making the right decision. I was listening to the experts and therefore this made me a good mum.

Taking the medication

The next morning I woke Seren up and it was the usual morning nightmare, which involved fighting with her to get her dressed, arguing with her to brush her teeth, or trying to get her to do anything that resembled getting ready for school. When she finally ate her breakfast, after three attempts, it was time for her to take the medication.

I found it ridiculous that we couldn't get Seren to follow a simple instruction and that something as simple as brushing her teeth could end up in the biggest fight ever, yet I was somehow supposed to get her to take a tablet. I ended up crushing it and putting it in a drink for her as there was no way that she was going to swallow the damn thing.

Seren finally took the medication, and conversations that I'd had with peers, pediatricians, psychologists and teachers started to swirl around my head.

'If she had diabetes then you would have to medicate her.'

'It's only the same as being diagnosed with an illness and then taking medication.'

'It's fine, you can't go on like this, you have made the right decision.'

When anyone tries to normalise the use of stimulant medication for children, they all seem to relate it to diabetes – why do they do this? They are not the same at all.

It took about forty minutes for the medication to take effect. After tormenting her brother and sister like she always did, and driving me around the bend, Seren then started to be kind to Daisy. We noticed the difference straightaway, as it was so rare. She then grabbed her bag, put on her school shoes and waited at the front door, something that she simply hadn't done before.

Daisy had started school a couple of weeks before the pediatrician diagnosed Seren. Daisy was only three but as she attended a Montessori school, children started school on the next term after their third birthday. Daisy, although only three years old, would grab her bag, put on her shoes and wait by the front door after we'd shout, 'Time to go to school'.

It would always amaze us that it could take fifteen minutes or more to get Seren to the front door, and yet Daisy would just wait there. It also confirmed to us that something was wrong with Seren, and it made us feel better about our decision to medicate, as we finally realised it wasn't down to 'bad parenting'. If we were bad parents, how could we have two children who acted so differently? How could Daisy respond so well to a request from Mummy and Daddy?

When it came to Seren, we would be screaming, at the end of our tether, and bright red with anger as she refused to put on her coat or put on her shoes!

The differences in my girls

This brings me to talk about the noticeable differences between Daisy and Seren. Daisy has always been tiny for her age, so she looks much younger than her years. Coupled with the fact that she was the sweetest, gentlest, most adorable three-year-old, it made everyone flock to her, especially the other kids at school.

I would pick Daisy up from school at 1.00 pm, which was also lunchtime for all the other kids, and they would run to Daisy (mainly the kids from Seren's class), circle her and want to cuddle her. They would take turns in picking her up and they all showered her with love and affection. Many of the girls adored Daisy and I guess that may have been quite hard on Seren. She was struggling to make new friends and Daisy was the most popular kid in the school.

Daisy, although she looked younger, has always seemed older than her years in the way she thinks. She remembers everything, is organised, and asks the most thought-out questions. 'Mummy, why is the sun following us?' 'Mummy, why does it rain?' 'Mummy, how can we get to the moon?' 'Mummy, who made this house and how did they do it?' Daisy's so intrigued with the way the world works, and has a presence that is pure and white; everyone around her feels it and people are drawn to her.

Daisy was born in caul, which means she was born in her amniotic sac. She was also born with a birthmark on the bottom of her back and one on her leg. The second midwife told us that being born 'in caul', along with her birthmarks, meant that Daisy was very spiritual. When I was pregnant with Daisy, I would play my HypnoBirthing music and lie under the trees to meditate. I would send love and kindness to Daisy. I would imagine the perfect birth in my mind over and over and I would tell myself how this was going to be a wonderful, calm birth free of fear and pain. Daisy's birth is still undoubtedly one of the most incredible memories of my life; everything that I had dreamt, imagined and visualised, came true.

I strongly believe in the power of the law of attraction. We can change our future through our thought patterns. If I truly believed in this statement, then what I was thinking, imagining and envisioning for Seren and her future, had to change.

Was it because of me?

My pregnancy with Seren wasn't bad, far from it, but I was in an entirely different place mentally. When I fell pregnant with Seren, I felt that she saved me. It felt like I was somehow putting the past behind me. I was excited about the new pregnant me, and a new baby; however, I do wonder whether how I was feeling at the time had any impact on Seren's behaviour. I was feeling very anxious when I conceived Seren and have always questioned whether the increase in cortisol could go through to the baby?

My life for the twelve months before I had Seren was pretty crazy. I was working in London, I had a major operation, got caught up in the London bombings, suffered from driving anxiety brought on by the London bombings, lost my licence through drink-driving caused by PTSD, got married, renovated two apartments, and then got pregnant.

To say my emotions, anxieties and fears were at fever pitch was an understatement! I did some research and found that there is evidence- based research on exactly this topic.

Many experts say that ADHD has nothing to do with the parents and there is nothing that we could have done to cause it, but I read a great book called the *ADHD Handbook*, which was written by an Australian psychologist, Stuart Passmore. He talks about ADHD in detail and also draws from his own experience as a psychologist. He was also the first person that I had come across to say that taking drugs or drinking heavily in pregnancy could cause ADHD.[11] I had never read this before and I started to worry about the glass of wine that I had when I was eight months pregnant with Seren! I will never know, but I am pretty sure that this wasn't the reason.

I am more concerned about how I was feeling throughout my pregnancy and how I felt in the months before I had Seren and whether it could have had an effect on her. If I believe that the relaxation, meditation, and the calm water birth, could have had a positive impact on Daisy and her personality, then surely how I felt months before I conceived Seren, her birth and the months after, could have impacted on her character. It takes me back to what I was saying before about Seren being made with 'too much cortisol'.

Back to medicating Seren

The first day that we medicated Seren, it was Karl who took the girls to school. He said Seren was fantastic all the way to the school. She did as she was told and was quiet and friendly to everyone (something that rarely happened), so we felt the medication was working.

I spoke to Seren's teacher later on that day and she felt that Seren had been really calm in school all day and had done lots of work. Slowly the guilt and anxiety started to fade; we must have made the right decision. The experts must have been right.

Later that night, she had a bath with her sister and was charming with her. For the first time, bath time didn't involve Daisy and Flynn screaming because Seren had taken all the room in the tub or splashed water at them or hurt them. It was all very calm, loving and relaxed. *Was this how it felt to be an ordinary family?*

Seren was usually like a jack-in-the-box, and having a bath meant throwing water all over the bathroom every time. It meant getting out of the tub and jumping on the bed, doing cartwheels, handstands, and pulling all the covers off the bed. Clothes would be flying everywhere. She would be screaming, giggling and chasing her siblings, but then she'd crash. Seren would be hysterical, fighting, wide-eyed, crying and shouting, and I could never believe how calm could turn to chaos in minutes and our nerves would be in tatters!

Well, this night wasn't like that at all. It was just like I'd imagined the perfect family bath time to be. How very Mary Poppins it seemed, as Seren did normal things like chat about her day and have a wash.

This drug was a miracle. Karl and I both felt so happy, we felt like we had made the right decision and our anxieties faded.

The next day was up and down and I remember feeling so confused as we'd had such a beautiful day with Seren the day before. This day, however, was very different to the previous. Seren was hyper and defiant.

Karl's mum, Mary, was arriving later that day and then Karl was going snowboarding for a week. It couldn't have come at a worse time for me, as

I knew that Mary didn't agree with ADHD or medicating children. With Karl leaving for a week, I was going to have to manage this on my own and I was starting to panic ...

Thank God for friends!

It was Sunday, and Karl was getting ready to go. Moments before he left, I opened my email and there were about ten emails from one of my best friends in the UK. Anna had been my confidant, along with my parents, and although she was 9,000 miles away, she had held my hand, listened to my problems and been there for me as I cried about our difficult situation with Seren.

Along with Anna, two of my good friends here in Perth were going through a similar thing with their daughter, but they were eighteen months ahead of us in the process, and like Anna they have been such incredible support.

No-one understands how you feel, or what it's like to be in this situation, unless they too are going through it themselves. And it's so true that you can never say what you would do or not do unless you are in that predicament yourself. How crazy it must have seemed, that someone who insisted on a natural way of living was now medicating her seven-year-old daughter. I was so embarrassed by who I had become. I felt lost and didn't recognise myself anymore.

Anna had told one of my other best friends, Olivia, that Seren was now being medicated with Ritalin. If we had been in the UK, I'm sure that Olivia would have popped over to see me as we had lived only miles apart. Instead, Olivia emailed me. She sent me lots of scary facts and figures about Ritalin and my heart totally and utterly sank, but I am grateful to her for standing up for something she believed in.

Correspondence during this time

18 August

Hi Susy,

I hope you don't mind but Anna told me about Seren being diagnosed with ADHD. I am worried about the drug Ritalin. I know you will have

50

researched this deeply but I am going to send you some information I have found. I hope you don't mind. Would love to have a chat with you too. Love you!
Love Olivia xx

Hey Olivia,

Thank you so much for this information. I will read it tonight/tomo and have a chat to Karl. We have started her on Ritalin as advised by her psychologist and pediatrician, but if there is another way I will take it with open arms.
We found an amazing difference in Seren for the first two days she was on the medication, but today we have had a hard day.
It's so hard to know what to do ... Thank you so much for sending me this. Things had got so bad. The school said most days she was so hyper they couldn't get her to do any work.
I will read it all, honey, and then give you a call. Thank you so much for caring.
Love Susy xx

Hi Susy,

Ahh my darling, I hope you're all ok. I know your children are your world and you would do anything for their best interests.
It must be so hard.
I know that Ritalin is an amphetamine, the same thing as speed. There is absolutely no difference. I will talk more when you have read what I have sent.
I also wanted you to know that I have only discussed this with Anna and Mark's sister. Anna only told me as she cares deeply about your situation and thinks it's good to see all sides.
I spoke to Mark's sister as I'm here with her all week and was interested in her thoughts.
Lots of love, Olivia xx

Hey Olivia,

Don't worry at all; I would have told you anyway. It's so hard to know what to do. Seren struggles so much as she is unable to concentrate at school. She's behind in her work and she's struggling to read. I am convinced that she has ADHD, but I'm not convinced by the Ritalin. It's so scary. She's been seeing a psychologist-play therapist for a couple of months now and she also feels that Ritalin is our only option. The school and pediatrician feel this too is the only answer.

I will read all the info though. Does Helen know of anything that can help? We've tried diet, fish oils ... therapy ... felt like this was the only way? Are you free to chat?

Love Susy xx

19 August

I am definitely around tomorrow, any time that suits you, honey. Talk to you tomorrow.

Love you x

Olivia x

Can't stop researching

I spent hours researching all the information that Olivia had sent me. I don't know why I hadn't read up on it all before; I was always Googling everything and anything, so why hadn't I done this?

If I am honest, it was because I knew it would be like this, and I was worried that all the scaremongering stories would stop me from medicating Seren. Karl and I promised each other that we wouldn't go to 'Dr Google' for advice, as you can never be sure what is accurate and what is false. We knew that this sort of information would completely freak us out, but here was one of my closest friends sending me this information, so it was something that I couldn't ignore.

When Seren was a baby, I discovered this amazing new world of baby groups and mothers meetings and I felt like it was my calling. Seven years later, I found this new world – the world of ADHD, but this was a much darker, scarier world – a world that I sometimes wish I had never discovered.

I found that doctors all over the Western world were diagnosing children with ADHD and subsequently medicating them with stimulant medication, often without looking at other possible factors. Once you are in the 'ADHD world' and on this path, for many, it gets darker and more medicated the longer you are on it.

What's so alarming is that in the process of writing this book, I went back to all the information that Olivia sent me, and much of it said how parents and teachers didn't know how to teach these hyperactive children and that medication had become too commonplace.

In my further research, I found that there are lots of pediatricians who are saving many families and suggesting other types of help such as occupational therapy, parenting methods and support from psychologists. However, many – if not most, certainly in Australia – are still adamant about using prescription medication to help with ADHD.

As I have said before, medication is helping many children and families all over the world. And many experts, teachers and parents will credit the use of stimulant medication in children. However, as ADHD is often mistaken for other symptoms, this could mean that children are being misdiagnosed and medicated with drugs that they don't need.

There also seems to be an increase in the amount of younger children who are being diagnosed and medicated, and this is also a very scary trend. And if I am brutally honest, if you have a pediatrician that suggests tests and supplements and maybe works with an occupational therapist, you have a pretty amazing one! Trying to find one like that, especially in countries like Australia and the US, is simply like trying to find unicorn shit!

Latest information from Australia states that many children are being medicated from the age of two, even though the latest 2012 National Health and Medical Research Council (NHMRC) Clinical Practice guideline states that, for children under seven, drugs should be the last resort. It is worrying that in the previous five years the number of children prescribed Ritalin between the ages 2–6 has gone up by 320%.[12]

I watched a documentary recently and it was all about the complexity of the brain, and even now we still don't understand its complexity or how to treat it for illnesses such as depression, bipolar or ADHD. If you go to the doctor and they suspect that you have diabetes, there are a range of blood tests and other tests that they will give you to determine the illness.

When you go to the doctor and they suspect you have depression, they give you a questionnaire to complete – or often they won't even do this, they will just prescribe antidepressants that come with a heap of side effects that often outweigh the medication benefits. But what if it wasn't depression in the first instance? What if Seren didn't have ADHD? What if we were all getting it so very wrong medicating such small, young, innocent minds with strong mind-altering drugs?

We all know that prescription medication has side effects, and for some children and families, not being medicated outweighs the side effects of being medicated. And for some families they have often tried everything and the only thing that works is medication. Or other parents welcome the diagnosis and are completely comfortable medicating their child in the first instance. That is their choice and if it's working for them, then amen to that.

The one thing I want to change – through writing this book – is the stigma and misunderstanding of ADHD. I want parents to be able to have conversations, to share information and to support each other. Many parents medicate; we have friends that medicate, and it doesn't mean that they love their child any less than we do. For them, after trying everything else, medication was the answer.

We live in a society where people are too quick to judge; you can't say anything these days without 'offending' people. I am not judging, and if you are reading this and you are medicating your child, please know that there is no judgement from me. I have been there and 'worn the t-shirt', as they say. I have been in your shoes.

We all just want our kids to be happy and to thrive in life, that's why we go to such lengths to try and fix them, make them fit in and make their little journeys in life as easy as possible. However, what I am saying is that there can be many variables that are not taken into consideration by the medical profession. They are too quick to diagnose and way too quick to medicate before even considering other things such as diet, deficiencies and other things that I will discuss further in the book.

When you are going through this as a parent, and there are millions of us who are, we often don't know where to turn. We are given so much conflicting advice – 'Shout at them and show them who's boss', 'Smack them, it never did me any harm', 'Just give them more love', 'It's your fault your daughter is frightened of you', 'She needs to show you more respect'.

It is never-ending.

We didn't tell Seren

We didn't tell Seren that she had been diagnosed with ADHD; we hadn't even convinced ourselves. It all happened so quickly, but I have since learnt that there are so many variables that could cause a child to be showing signs of ADHD. Diet, allergies, sugar, toxins, metals, abuse or addiction in the family, hearing problems, trauma, PTSD, the list is endless but the diagnosis is always the same – 'ADHD'.

It has now become the 'one size that fits all' diagnosis, which isn't affected by race or social status – everyone from every household and walk of life is now affected by ADHD and its over-diagnosis.

Do you have a child that can't sit still? ADHD.

Do you have a child that interrupts when you are speaking? ADHD.

Do you have a child that is behind in school? ADHD.

Do you have a child that can't concentrate? ADHD.

Do you have a child that runs off and doesn't obey instructions? ADHD every time.

And be careful which psychologist you see as you could find yourself – the parent – also being labelled with 'ADHD' and prescribed Ritalin. BOOM! Another score for the pharmaceutical companies!

I have also thought it is so odd that boys were more likely to have ADHD than girls. Everyone knows that they run, climb trees, flight, play, and are full-on compared to girls who like to sit and play with dolls, play mummies and daddies, and wear pink tutus. I am over generalising here, but you get the gist!

Could it be that childhood has now become a symptom of ADHD and that we are simply 'medicating childhood'? These were just some of the thoughts I had whirling around my head as we tried to deal with our situation.

More and more findings ...

More recently, though, I read some information about the studies of Dr Nicole Brown, who feels that childhood trauma could be mistaken for ADHD, and how we are too quick to medicate. One in nine US children, or 6.4 million, are currently diagnosed with ADHD.[13]

There have also been similar studies by Dr Kate Symanski, who also linked abuse, neglect and household dysfunction to ADHD, and questioned if it was ADHD or something else, and whether pediatricians were too quick to medicate without properly assessing the children first.[13]

Dr Brown goes on to say that, in recent years, parents and experts have questioned whether the growing prevalence of ADHD has to do with hasty medical evaluations, a flood of advertising for ADHD drugs, and increased pressure on teachers to cultivate high-performing students.[13]

I have to say that given my experience over the last eighteen months, it would be irresponsible and unfair to our children of the world today if we didn't realise that this statement was 100% true. I will come to this in more detail later on in this book, but if Seren did have ADHD, then how could she be such a different child without medication eighteen months later?

At one point, Seren's behaviour was so bad that I was starting to think the devil possessed her, and I even found myself Googling 'devil possession'. Eighteen months later, she is just an ordinary kid. Yes, she is hyper, forgetful, over-emotional and challenging at times. Inattentive is still her 'middle name', but I wouldn't even consider medication now. For us, the side effects outweighed the benefits, but the drugs also changed her personality and I hated that. We have now learnt to love so many of her quirky little layers, and medication would only drown out some of her strengths as well as her weaknesses.

Stopping the medication

After reading all the information that Olivia had sent me, I was so petrified by it all that we decided to stop Seren taking medication straightaway. Yes, we had seen positive results – her behaviour was better and her teacher had confirmed that Seren's behaviour had been much better.

But after reading all the frightening information, there was absolutely no way that I could give this to Seren unless I knew I had tried absolutely every other single thing known to man. So, with my mother-in-law staying and Karl gone for the week, I had to manage this on my own, which scared the living daylights out of me.

One of the things that Seren doesn't cope well with is change, and Daddy going on holiday for a week was never going to be easy. Karl's mum, Mary, has always been extremely close to Seren and our family, so it must have been very hard for her to accept the changes that were taking place with Seren's behaviour, and also for her to accept this very sudden diagnosis and medication plan.

Diary entries during this time

4 August

I had one of the worst weeks ever with Seren. Mary witnessed Seren's constant outbursts, observed my haphazard responses and probably noted that my relationship with Seren was non-existent. I know that I was showing more love towards Daisy and Flynn, but I just didn't know how to change it. Lucy was here too with the twins. I totally lost it at bath time and started to shout at Seren. They can see I am not coping. I hate myself.

12 August

I still feel very depressed! I can't think straight, don't want to leave the house! I feel awful today!

My day was ok in the end. Had a nice night with Seren. Sometimes I honestly find it hard to cope with the kids. It's so full-on – sometimes it's like torture!

Ups and downs, ups and downs

Only towards the end of the journey would I come to realise that Seren didn't play up on purpose, she wasn't being vindictive or evil, or trying to 'wind me up'. To be honest, she didn't even have the capability to think like that; however, when you are in it at the time, you would swear that your child was misbehaving just to upset you!

I have learnt so much on this journey, and I have learnt that it's not about me anymore – it's about Seren. I must stop taking it so personally, it's just the way Seren is, it's the way she's made, it's her personality, and shouting, smacking and medicating isn't going to make a blind bit of difference.

Seren is Seren – the end.

Seren's behaviour now doesn't bother me (ok, I am not always able to say that). Yes, it's hard and it takes its toll at times. I have had to learn to the have the patience of a saint; in fact, my patience now makes the patience of a saint look pathetic. I mean I would literally blow them out of the water in the 'patience competition'!

I don't take it personally anymore and I realise it's not a personal attack against me. I have come to understand that it's not her fault, she's not bad, defiant or naughty; she can't help it.

I know there is a fine line, but if I cross it, the only person that I hurt is myself.

However, I didn't know any of this at the time, so my relationship with Seren was in tatters. She would play up, and I would get angry. She would become more defiant, and I would get even angrier – and so it would continue.

Seren would see that I was angry and then she would start screaming and so it would go on until Seren would run out of the house into the street screaming. I can only imagine what the neighbours must have thought. It used to break our hearts; Seren would be screaming and shouting at us, and then she would run out of the house, often in her underwear, still screaming and yelling. I would run to her and try and get her to come back into the house, and then as I would get close, she would run again. It was literally soul destroying. She seemed so scared, so out of control, so lost, that I feared the worst.

Although at times I shouted and screamed at her, very often, I would be quite calm. Seren wasn't smacked or abused or locked in her room, but if you were a neighbour and you heard the constant, daily screaming, you would have thought that much worse was going on.

Maybe she does need medication?

One day, Nana (Mary) said she would take Seren to school. Now, to most children this would be exciting, and although Seren was hugely excited, it was also a 'change'. Seren didn't 'do' change!

The morning that Nana was going to take Seren to school, Seren had said she didn't like her hair and asked if I would do it again. I explained that she was late for school and that I couldn't. And that was it – Seren became aggressive, violent, angry, and she started screaming and running around. It ended with Seren hiding in the garage, with me trying to grab her out from behind the bikes. The bikes then started falling on top of Seren and she started screaming so loud that I worried about what the neighbours thought of me. 'Leave me alone, don't come near me, get away from me,' she screamed.

I looked at Mary and noticed that she was crying. I saw the pain in her eyes and I could see this was breaking her heart – it was breaking mine too, I just didn't know what to do. Seren got out from underneath the bikes, pushed past me and Mary, and then ran out of the garage, through the house and out of the front door. I watched as she vanished down the road. *Why did this happen? Why was she acting like a crazy child? What was going on? Maybe she did need the medication? What have I done?*

Mary finally managed to get Seren to come back home and go to school that day, but not until much later. Mary and I were physically and emotionally drained – what we had witnessed just wasn't normal and we were both so scared. Mary didn't mention anything when she got back from taking Seren to school that morning. I desperately wanted to talk to her about what had happened, but I could see it was too painful. I called Seren's teacher and explained that Seren had a terrible morning and asked her to please keep an eye on her and let me know if she was ok–I was out of mind with worry. I couldn't believe that this two-hour ordeal all happened because I said I didn't have time to put a bun in her hair.

Correspondence during this time

20 August

Hi Susy,
All is ok, don't worry. I will keep an eye on Seren. We have had a chat and I explained that if she wanted to have a co-worker, she needed to be quiet and still, and friendly so that a good working relationship could occur. We observed other pairs of working children and I stressed the point that all of these partners were working calmly and with purpose. A friend offered to work with Seren, so I will keep them on track and hopefully her day will be full and happy.
Yesterday, Seren wanted to get up and down a lot, and even though she was assigned a desk, other children ebbed and flowed around her with purpose and were oblivious to her social needs because they were happy just getting their work done.
I know that work and focus will ground her agitation and the social network will flow when that comes more naturally.
Have a lovely day.

Diane xx

Hi Diane,

Thank you so much for your continued support. Karl is away until tomorrow, but I feel it might be a good idea to try her on the Ritalin again while we explore other avenues. I will have a good talk to Karl when he gets back.

I don't think I've ever been faced with such a difficult decision, Diane, in my whole life!

Thank you so much for everything.

Love Susy xx

I felt like a rabbit in the headlights; I was frozen with fear, panicking and not coping. I couldn't stop thinking about the conflicting advice on ADHD. How could one group of professionals support medication and then another group of professionals slander it? The information that Olivia had sent me included statements from professionals (world-leading psychiatrists, psychologists, pediatricians, teachers and parents) that said the use of Ritalin in children was wrong. There was so much negative information out there. I once typed into Google, 'Ritalin ruined my life', and what I read was harrowing!

I was lost and frightened and I missed Karl so much. These were decisions that I didn't want to make by myself anymore.

Mary, although she didn't agree with Ritalin, gave me her blessing to try it again on Seren. I knew what a big thing this was for her, as she didn't agree with medicating children. However, Mary could see how this was destroying our family and she could see how troubled Seren was. I did consider it again, but questioned how I could give her something that had so many side effects and such negative propaganda. I hated this situation. I wanted it to stop. I just wanted to go back to the way things were, at least before the diagnosis.

We had previously thought it was just bad behaviour and we were managing it (even if it was crisis management). I desperately wanted to go back to those days; however, we couldn't, we were in it – hook, line and sinker – and there was no going back.

Chapter Four

Homeopaths, naturopaths and different paths

When did life become so complex and sophisticated? I was brought up with jam sandwiches, fizzy lemonade, bike rides until dusk, and muddy knees. I never heard my mother mention the words – anxiety, folate, leaky gut, gluten-free or defective genes. Have we all gone slightly mad and it's now our children who are paying the price?

Karl came home and Mary went to stay with Karl's brother, so there was a bit of normality at home again. Normality and routine always meant that Seren's behaviour would be slightly better. She simply couldn't cope with change. If the slightest things were different in school or at home, Seren's behaviour would start to become very challenging.

Sometimes when Seren was younger, if someone popped around unannounced, Seren's demeanour would take a nosedive. She would start shouting at everyone, scowl at the person who came into the house and immediately would start being mean to me and shouting at me.

We would always feel totally embarrassed and felt like people must have thought that manners and good behaviour didn't matter in our house, when they actually meant so much. Again, I have learnt that often ADHD children aren't good with change or transition, so going to different places, or someone popping around unannounced, can send them into a spin. However, this 'spin' was never a cute little spin – it was more like an 'angry, fierce house-ripping up tornado' type spin!

Off to the naturopath we go

One of the great things about Perth is that it has an abundance of naturopaths. I had never come across a naturopath before and I wasn't even sure what they did.

This was the start of the never-ending appointments that I went along to with Seren. But I was determined to find a more natural way to do things.

At this point we were told that ADHD was a disorder or a disease. We were told that it wasn't down to diet or parenting, so if that was true then surely I could find a 'cure'. I was feeling extremely confident. I had read many ADHD books and I spent so much time researching ADHD on Google, but there was still so much more information to read and look through. I didn't know where to start, so I was hoping that the natural doctors could help me.

Naturopathy is a holistic approach to wellness; it treats each person as an individual and supports the whole person to live a healthier lifestyle. The foundations of naturopathy are based on the importance of a healthy diet; fresh, clean water; sunlight; exercise, and stress management. Surely if I worked on all these things, this would help Seren's ADHD.

Naturopathy aims to educate the person (or parents) to look after their health and the health of their family, minimising symptoms of any illness, supporting the body's capacity to heal, and balancing the body so that illness is less likely to occur in the future.[14]

It all sounded very la-di-da, happy and healthy!

While chatting to the naturopath, she explained that we needed to immediately take dairy and gluten out of Seren's diet. At the time of seeing the naturopath, we were all vegetarians, although we had recently started eating fish. She went on to explain how children needed meat, especially red meat that contained iron, and she told me that low iron could cause behavioural problems in children.

I wondered why the pediatrician hadn't taken any blood tests before handing out medication so quickly; surely they should check these sorts of things before so readily diagnosing Seren with ADHD? Anyway, none of that mattered anymore; we were in good hands and surely everything would be ok now...

The naturopath arranged for Seren to have some blood tests so she could check Seren's iron levels along with zinc, magnesium, vitamin D, vitamin B and other such things. She felt that if Seren was low in vital vitamins and minerals, this could be affecting her behaviour. She also gave me some tests that I had to do at home.

A friend, whose daughter had ADHD, told me that nutrition is often underplayed in ADHD management, but there are nutritional deficiencies that appear in most cases of ADHD children. There is a link between children with ADHD and low iron but they don't know what the link is. I'm no expert, but wouldn't it be better for the child to be given iron, vitamins and supplements before medicating them with stimulant medication?

The naturopath told me that stimulant medication could actually cause the body to become even more depleted in vital vitamins and minerals.

Nutritional deficiencies

A lot of the deficiencies that Seren had are critical in the neurotransmitter balance. The most common nutritional deficiencies in ADHD children include low B vitamin levels, low magnesium, along with low zinc and low fatty acids.[15] There are other things as well, but I will get to them later.

We also needed to check to see if Seren had a defective gene. The naturopath explained that if Seren was low in this particular folate, also named the MTHFR gene, this could be linked to ADHD-type symptoms. And if Seren had this defective gene and other deficiencies, the worst thing we could do to her was to medicate her with a stimulant-based drug.

The gut!

The naturopath also talked about gut health and how important this was for everyone, but especially children. She told me that gut health is as important as mental health and that experts now realise that our serotonin levels are in our gut. I had never heard this before, and like most things on this journey it fascinated me, so of course I went home and Googled it!

I don't know what I would have done without the internet, it has helped me so much. I have a love/hate relationship with it, and at times I have loathed what I've read about ADHD. It has brought me to tears, but on other occasions I have had so many 'light bulb' moments that I have wanted to shout it from the rooftops. I guess that's why I started to write this book, maybe this way I could shout it from the rooftops, but in a different way, through words in a book.

I found out that the gut is created from the same tissue as the brain during foetal development, and that experts are now realising that our happiness depends on the health of your digestive tract, where at least 80% of our serotonin supply is manufactured.[16]

80%. That's huge!

Why are they still treating people with drugs for the brain if most of the serotonin is in the gut?

I have always laughed to Karl that many experts aren't 100% sure that a child has ADHD when they medicate them, but they feel that because they are displaying so many of the symptoms, the medication should fix the problem.

It's like saying, 'We think your leg has gangrene, we aren't 100% sure, but just to cover all options, we are going to remove it anyway'. I joke here, but mental health is no laughing matter and it should be taken as seriously as the health of our body. Just because we can't see it, it doesn't mean it's not as important. It needs to be dealt with correctly, not by just throwing something at it and hoping for the best.

Seren's diet

I went away with my blood test forms, two other types of tests that we had to do at home, and some fascinating information that I had to think on.

The naturopath continually talked about diet, so we went through Seren's diet. Although she praised me for it being healthy, she went on to explain that it was high in gluten and dairy and gave me a brief overview of how this affects the gut and therefore a child's behaviour. The naturopath told me how this is linked to 'leaky gut syndrome'. This is a phrase that I am reading a lot about now.

I had spent the last four months researching ADHD; I had read all about the symptoms, the causes and the alternative treatments. I had signed up for a parenting course, added myself to so many different ADHD newsletters that I had lost count, and now this – leaky gut syndrome!

Serotonin in the gut, deficiencies, gluten-free, dairy-free, and what on earth was MTHFR all about? My head raced around continually with all these thoughts, and for the first time I stopped Googling 'ADHD' (for now anyway).

Correspondence and diary entries during this time

30 August

Hi Diane,

I just wanted to let you know that Seren had some marine phytoplankton before school today (as you do). It's supposed to help with concentration, so please let me know if you notice any difference this week. I will keep you posted about the other stuff, but I've got a clear plan now of which way to go with it all.

Thanks so much, Diane. I would also like to take the opportunity to thank you so much for all your help and support with Seren. She is very lucky to have such a wonderful teacher.

Kind regards, Susy xx

31 August

Hi Susy,

Thanks for the kind message.

Today I limited Seren's movements and asked that she choose a desk to work from, as she was not settling as well as the other children. She wanted to do lots of things but was not accomplishing one thing at a time.

Having one space and being monitored helped her stay on track.

I will continue to do this, as she is unable to cope with the freedom of wide-open spaces and free choice. This is a common technique for attention enhancement. It will help her improve her executive functioning skills so that when I see she can cope, we will widen the perimeters of choice and space.

She got a lot more done than yesterday. Her memory retention requires focus now, so can you see how she goes with reading practice tonight.

Diane xx

3 September

I haven't updated this for a while; however, as per the naturopath, I have taken gluten and dairy out of Seren's diet. We have been doing this for about two weeks and I have noticed a remarkable difference. Mornings this week and last week were better. Seren was really good getting ready, and the mornings were calmer.

The week before was a challenge – changing clothes and hairstyles before school, slamming doors and gates. :-(

We are also giving Seren zinc, magnesium, fish oils and iron. She eats gluten-free and dairy-free and we have now started giving her meat, which she has at lunchtime.

I have been to LADS, which supports parents with ADHD children here in Perth. They have told me about a behavioural model/chart to use, so we will be implementing it this week.

She has been for a mauve and MTHFR test and I will get the results in a week. She will also be tested for metals and have an intolerance/allergy test.

4 September

We went to a seminar with Dr Stephen Hughes, who talked at length about executive functioning and ADHD. He also talked about Ritalin and how it increases the dopamine that is lacking in ADHD children.

I feel that since taking gluten/dairy out, there has been an improvement. I spoke with Seren's teacher today and sadly there has been no difference there. She is still unable to concentrate in school.

I am reading the ADHD Handbook and it talks about ADHD and the fact that it is over-diagnosed.

Is she suffering from anxiety? The move? Loss of friends?

I'm seeing the psychologist in two weeks. We can then formulate a plan – we can discuss this at length.

Will also start the chart tomorrow for both girls, as Daisy's behaviour is changing. Is she copying Seren? Is it her age?

Four months in

It's interesting that four months into our ADHD journey with Seren, I asked myself these questions – was it anxiety, the move, loss of friends?

All the experts thought not, but looking back now I can see that this had an impact on Seren, and I have since learnt that many different environmental factors have an effect on a child's behaviour. Children are not as resilient as we think they are. They are not able to process things as adults do – realising that they are stressed and then sitting down to rationalise it all.

They are children. Even as adults, we are still not able to always do this, which is why I believe so many people are on medication for depression and anxiety.

I only learnt all this as I was going through the journey with Seren. At the age of thirty-nine, I have finally come to understand why I sometimes felt anxious, depressed, and acted the way I did. I only wish that I'd been taught about self-regulation and emotional intelligence in school, or by my parents, when I was younger (I'm not even sure it was around then). Remember that most of us in the 70s and 80s were brought up on jam sandwiches for lunch. Life was so much simpler.

Life is pretty easy for some

Another thing that I have learnt is that if you are like Karl or Daisy, then life is pretty easy. They are calm, rational, and consistent. They move slower, and they consider their surroundings. They are happy, relaxed, and I would love to live in their bodies and minds for just one hour to see what it's like!

Once on holiday, while I was looking out to sea with Karl, holding hands and feeling so happy at that moment, I asked Karl what he was thinking. He said, 'Nothing, I just appreciate how beautiful this moment is, and how breathtaking the ocean is ...' Or something like that anyway.

I couldn't believe it! Nothing, I mean, nothing? How is that even possible?

He asked me what I was thinking, and although I can't exactly remember what I said, it went something like this:

'Wow, look how amazing the ocean is. I wonder what creatures are swimming in the ocean right now? There must be so many beautiful fish out there. Fish, I can't believe I ate fish yesterday, I'm supposed to be a vegetarian. I have been a vegetarian for a long time, and I'm breastfeeding Flynn, and he feeds a lot, and I'm super tired. I might go for a nap after this. I love being with Karl. I love him. Daisy and Seren, where are they? Oh, there they are, all good. God, I am exhausted. I might get a coffee, oh no I'm breastfeeding, and I've already had two coffees today. I will get an ice-cream, though, but I'm still overweight. Susy, it's fine, you have a small baby and you are breastfeeding. Yes, that's right, I deserve an ice-cream. Oh wow, look how big those waves are ...'

I kid you not. That all probably happened in a few seconds. Karen says that when she is sitting with me, she reckons she can hear the 'cogs turning'. Thinking, planning, plotting and sorting everything and anything all in one little moment while having a cuppa and chat on a sunny afternoon.

I can't help it, and Seren is the same. We are hyperactive, talkative, excitable, nervous, angry, anxious, giggly, emotional and clumsy, and life can often seem harder. It's a challenge to stay happy, positive and focused as you are in a constant battle with your monkey brain, which is forever running away with itself! However, with that comes passion, creativity, kindness, laughter, and love, so I have learnt to go with it, work on the anger and impulsivity, meditate, exercise, eat well, drink less coffee and alcohol and walk – walking is so good for the mind, body and soul (oh yes, I must remember to walk more).

For me, I know that the only time my mind is quiet is when I ride my bike. *Do I ride my bike often?* No, but I should and it's definitely on the list! The list that is never-ending – that unattainable bloody list – now where is that list?

It took me almost forty years to realise that I probably have ADHD too. I have never been diagnosed, but I tick every box! Although, as I have got older, it's been much easier to manage. Suddenly my haphazard, impulsive, crazy twenties all made perfect sense.

I will discuss this in more detail later on. However, I want to ensure that this book it about Seren's journey, not my own, but my journey may help other parents who are struggling with ADHD themselves.

Blood tests

As instructed by the naturopath, I took Seren to the doctors to have a blood test. It's important to mention here that trying to get Seren to have a blood test was like trying to get a square peg through a round hole. There were so many tantrums, screaming fits and tears that I thought it would never happen. The impossible act of trying to get an over-emotional, hyperactive, defiant seven-year-old to allow the doctor to insert a needle and draw blood seemed as big as climbing Everest!

But, in the end, a visit to the toy shop first, bribery, sweets, a book to read while we there, prayers and lots of crossing fingers and toes, Seren had the blood test. However, afterwards she screamed like someone had just chopped her leg off without anaesthesia!

The results came back and Seren was low in iron, vitamin D, which is funny as that's from sunlight and we live in Australia (now we always do the ten minutes in the sun without sunscreen rule). She was also low in zinc and magnesium, so the naturopath gave me some supplements for Seren, as well as some herbs.

The tests also concluded that Seren had a faulty MTHFR gene and that she would need some supplements and vitamins to support this. Apparently, this is when your body isn't able to use folate properly, which is vitamin B9.

To be honest, I didn't take it seriously at the time and it's only since writing this book that I have decided to have a closer look at this, and see if there is something more that can be done to help Seren.

Diary entries during this time

5 September

Seren woke up and started being mean to Daisy and Flynn. She demanded that everyone get out of the bedroom, even though I was in my own room feeding Flynn. I sent her out after she told me that she hated me. She calmed down and was fine. I had to collect her from school as she wasn't well. It was the easiest night I have ever had as she slept all day and night.

6 September

Seren has been amazing today; she is just so well behaved. We spent three hours doing craft today and then went to the shops and she was so good. She is being beautiful with Daisy and Flynn, and is just so calm. Billy, Lucy and the twinnies came to stay as Karl is away and they noticed how amazing she was too! :-)

7 September

Wow, the best behaviour I've ever had – obedient, gracious, kind, amazing! What is happening? Her reading isn't going very well, though, but it's so much better. I've had the most wonderful weekend with her. I'm calm, though, so is it that? :-)

8 September

Seren woke up unwell and I couldn't get her out of bed. I felt she was pretending, as she had been fine all weekend. I was sure that this would turn out badly!

It didn't though and she got dressed, had her breakfast and got into the car! She also played craft with Daisy in school today (Montessori allow children to have lunch dates with each other's classes).

It was difficult going to bed, as she was so hyper! I think there is a link with tomatoes. Overall, very impressed with her behaviour.

9 September

Seren has been more challenging today. She has been running off, walking off in a mood and being bad tempered. I have to repeat myself over and over. It's time to do the chart! I am doing it tomorrow night that is for sure!

10 & 11 September

Seren's behaviour is starting to change ... It's the time of the month for me, so is it that? She's not listening again, being defiant, mean with her sister and brother. The impulsivity is back and she kicked Flynn in the head. She has started running off to the neighbour's house again without asking and knocking on their door.

I spoke with her teacher and she advised me that she allows Seren to do something that she loves, which then increases the dopamine, and then she can manage to get her work done as she can focus more.

I'm upset as I feel she has gone backwards. Maybe it's because I haven't been able to spend as much time with her because Karl is away?

She hasn't been eating her meat at lunchtime either – I am exhausted with it all, to be honest. Karl is back and I'm already noticing a change for the worse. Must do the chart!!!!!!!!!!!

Too much going on

When I read those diary entries now, I don't actually think Seren's behaviour seems so terrible. But, what is interesting is that like most mothers who are going through this, you are already at the end of your tether and your cup is full! Your cup is so full that it's bubbling and frothing and spilling all over the table.

You are stressed, you are sad, you are bewildered, and you are like a moth that keeps touching the light. It burns every time but you can't stop going towards it, so you go back and forth, back and forth, in a stressed blizzard of chaos.

What's so clear to me now as I read these diary entries is that Seren couldn't handle change. Karl at the time was travelling more than usual, so the change of him going away, then being away, and then coming back, for Seren, was a game changer. Even though the teacher and the psychologist had mentioned it to me, I didn't appreciate how much bearing it had on Seren's mood and personality.

The complexities of the behavioural chart

What's also interesting to note is that I keep talking about the behavioural chart, but I never, ever did it. *Why?* Honestly, it was way too confusing, and with an ADHD child, a toddler, a baby, and Karl away a lot, I needed a quick fix and the behavioural chart sent my head into a spin.

The psychologist told me to ignore the bad and praise the good, but at the time, this was so hard as Seren seldom did anything good. She would spend all day being mean to the family, running off, being defiant, not getting dressed, refusing to eat her breakfast; it went on and on, how on earth could I ignore all that and only focus on the good?

They also said we had to give her praise as soon as she did something good and then give her something tangible, as ADHD kids have to see and feel it, they simply couldn't understand that they would receive something later. I asked her for ideas on this, but she didn't give me any, she just said it had to be 'instant'. *What is instant?* I certainly couldn't give her sweets (they made her crazy), she wasn't bothered by food, money or material things, so what was I supposed to give her?

The support worker at the ADHD centre in Perth had also talked about a reward system; she talked about something with coloured plastic tokens, colour-coded for different things that would apply to our family. For instance, we could give Seren a blue token when she got dressed, which was worth one point; a green token for listening to Mummy, which was worth two points; and a red token for not running off, which was the holy grail as this gave Seren three points!

This would be accompanied by a wall chart that would list all the things that I wanted Seren to do: get dressed, eat breakfast, be kind, listen to Mummy, etc. Seren could colour it and then I would need to make sure that I had a never-ending supply of blue, green and red tokens – remembering to have them at home, in the car and my bag – while always remembering to ignore the bad and focus on the good!

The whole thing filled me with dread! We had tried so many behaviour charts over the years and Seren had always proceeded to rip them off the wall, tear them up and sometimes even put them in the bin! Seren would take anything from anywhere so I could imagine me shouting at her, 'Where are the tokens that were in my bag?' Or, 'Seren, why have you got a collection of tokens in your room under your pillow?'

I saw myself out at the park, thinking, *damn I forgot those bloody tokens again and Seren has just been kind to her brother, hang on was it green or red for kindness*? And just as I was about to go over and give her hug and tell her that I owed her a red token (as I had forgotten them again), she would kick her sister in the head ... so, what happens then? Do I take the red token away? *Do I ignore the kick in the head and still give her the token from the cuddle she just gave her brother*?

Are you as confused as me? It makes me laugh just thinking about it, and this was the reason that despite all my 'must do the chart tomorrow' entries, I have never actually got around to doing it! I was so confused and bewildered that I never even printed the chart off, or bought the tokens because clearly there is a blue, green and red token shop somewhere surely?

Honestly, I don't mean to be unkind but I didn't find the advice from the 'ADHD support group' helpful at all. The lady advised me that she was a volunteer and I commend her for trying to help so many parents and children, but I left that day feeling more confused than ever. She did give me some great handouts and they did tell me that anxiety can be linked to ADHD, but they didn't say anything about diet, supplements, etc. that I have since found out are the absolute foundation of helping your child to thrive with ADHD.

I have since made up my own reward system that is so easy, simple and efficient! Never mind the 'behaviour chart', they've got nothing on my system! All I use is a jam jar and some coins and it's the best thing I have ever used. It's easy to use as a parent, and it's easy for the kids to understand. I don't need to remember anything when I am out, there is no chart, no fuss and it's positive reinforcement. I only wish I had discovered it years ago! It's very similar to the 'pasta in the jar' method that Karl's Auntie Carol told me about a few years before, but I slightly tweaked it.

I filled the jar with 10 cents to the value of $5. Every time Seren would do something out of line – for example: refusing to get dressed for school, brush her teeth, tidy her room, or if she would do something like scream or slam a door, run off, whatever it was – I would take a coin out of the jar.

I would immediately say to Seren that I would put the money back in the jar as soon as she did the task or changed her behaviour. As soon as I would see her show kindness to her siblings, put on her shoes, tidy up or get dressed, the money would go back into the jar.

I would always make sure that when I took money out, I would assure her that the money would go back in once she did something well. And so, Seren would be continually trying to do something well to get the money back in the jar.

I would use this method while we were out at the park or even on holiday, even though there was visually no jar or money; I guess in these situations it was more about positive reinforcement.

The aim of the process was to keep all the money in the jar by Friday, and then it would be treat night. For Seren, this meant pizza, popcorn and a movie – this to her was perfection! The money didn't matter really, it was just a visual aid and a sort of incentive that keeping the money in the jar by Friday would mean that she would get her reward (how great it would be if pizza, popcorn and a movie did only cost $5). You can use anything though – dried pasta, money, buttons, or get yourself some of those tokens from the token shop that's around somewhere!

Diary entries during this time

18 September
Still very hyper! We have stopped the herbs as they seem to make her more hyper, and we have also stopped the vitamins for the folate thingy, as again they appear to make her very hyper. But I am not sure if it is that, it's so hard to know! Anyway, I am just going to carry on giving her the zinc, magnesium, fish oils and the homoeopathy and see how it goes.

Her teachers have noticed that she is very hyper too. I honestly feel desperate at this stage! We have taken out food groups, given her supplements, and none of it seems to work for long. She is starting to read though, which is good. Her teacher doesn't think she is dyslexic, she just thinks she can't remember words! Anyway, going to book the IQ test and see what happens with this. I feel so stressed with it all; I honestly don't know what to do!
:-(HELP!!!!!!!!!!!!!

I am feeling so stressed today with it all. I miss people, miss my friends and my family, could do with a good girly chat!

I feel so alone and confused. I am meeting with the psychologist next week, hoping this will help!

21 September

Going to start the homoeopathic treatments today! Definitely not the herbs, they seem to make her hyper!!! Going to watch the TV program called *Kids on Speed* that my friend told me about and then start the behaviour chart!

22 September

Karl said Seren was fantastic last night – reading, helping and calm. She had her homoeopathy this morning, so now that we have taken out the herbs we can monitor this and see if there is a change.

She helped at breakfast this morning, got dressed, played nicely with her siblings and then read amazingly well. She hugged me, promised to be a good girl in school and then left smiling. What is happening? She was so loving with Daddy last night too!

23–25 September

Seren was fantastic, getting her clothes ready for school the night before in neat piles, being amazing in the morning. Great at school – perfect!

27 September

We had to stay in the house today and we have found it tough. She was very impulsive, hyper, hitting, screaming at Flynn. She starting pouring water all over the kitchen floor and walls – we have been really busy today, so was it that? I haven't been able to give her a lot of attention.

She does seem very hyper. I forgot to give her her homoeopath this morning, so maybe it's that?

29 September
Terrible behaviour!!!! Defiant, running away, hyper, naughty. God, it's been such a hard day. Is it the gluten? I am exhausted!

30 September
Seren is still being full-on, but I have to say after the homoeopathic treatment she was amazing! Overall she has been tough today. Hyper, defiant, running off out of the restaurant! The homoeopathist told me to give Seren the remedy every other day, but I'm thinking maybe we will do it every day, as there is a difference in her behaviour when she doesn't have it.

3 October
Definitely more defiant than usual, and hyper. I am finding it harder to control her diet as she is refusing to eat meat or non-dairy and non-gluten foods!
The homoeopathy is helping, though. We are going on holiday so I am packing, is it that? We got to the airport and Seren was difficult, running off, defiant, even the airport staff were getting annoyed with her! Sometimes I wonder if life would be easier with Ritalin???? But then I have a word with myself and man up!!!

Holidays, or 'hell-i-days'

We had been trying natural alternatives for two months; it was now October and we were going on a road trip from Cairns to Brisbane for Karl's 40th birthday.

We were going to spend three weeks in a camper van and then fly to Bali for a week to join Karl's brother and his family. I was so excited by the whole thing, we all were. However, I look back now and I start to hyperventilate when I even think of the trip.

We have always tried to live a normal life, even though we have had a challenging child, whom we have since realised DOES NOT COPE WITH CHANGE! But I was determined that this wouldn't stop us from getting out and about. We couldn't just live our lives in the house, not going on holidays, not going out for day trips or having people over for ... dare I say it ... 'a coffee and catch up'!

Seren absolutely has to be in control, she can't help it. Even going somewhere different for a day out, or breakfast, can literally tip her over the edge. However, now that we can recognise it, we reassure her, hug her, make her feel safe and loved.

And how do I know this? Because I get like that too!

The psychologist had said to me that ADHD kids don't like change. However, at the time, Seren's behaviour was pulling me deep into the quicksand so fast that I couldn't breathe, I just couldn't see it!

Constantly during the holiday, I found myself saying to Karl:

'She's so naughty.'

'She just wants her own way.'

'She will learn to do as she's told.'

'She never listens.'

'I will not put up with this anymore, she will do as she is told while she lives under our roof!' (Or to be more specific, the tiny campervan that we were all squeezed into, roof!)

Honestly, some of the things I used to say I could hear my dad's voice coming out of my mouth – these were his words, not mine! Have you ever noticed that you can say things and then you realise that you were told those exact things as a kid? And did they work? No!

I remember at age three, my dad was screaming at me, 'Susy if you do that again, you will get a mighty one'. (Just to confirm, a 'mighty one' was pants down and many smacks on the bottom.) I remember it vividly. I would then plead, 'I didn't mean to do that or say that, please can I have another chance', but it was too late and so Dad would charge over to grab me (gulp). If I knew that I would get a mighty one, and I knew that it would hurt, why would I not just do as I was told? My dad would also hang my 'Gee Gee' (AKA security blanket) on the bannister, leaving my bedroom door open so I could see Gee Gee hanging there. I would cry for Gee Gee and desperately want to hug him as I lay there with a stinging red bottom. *Why oh why did I never learn?*

I can remember this so clearly, and I was only three. I don't know why I did it, though. Daisy and Flynn don't do it. I can ask them to stop doing something and mostly they will, or at least they will stop after a second time when I politely ask them to stop.

But Seren, she has that 'inner naughty monster' inside her just like I did, only now the experts tell us it's 'impulsivity', but is it really? Or is it just a 'naughty monster' and we have all gone slightly mad trying to label every child that is impulsive, hyper or out of control.

During this holiday (um, I mean road trip hell as we now remember it), I didn't remember what I was like at three. I didn't think of Seren's behaviour as a cute little naughty monster with googly eyes. Oh no, I believed that Seren was a crazed, wild lunatic, and as soon as we got home we would go and see somebody, anybody, who could help us with this situation.

We were definitely still not coping!

Diary entries during this time

4 October
We arrived in Cairns and Seren was very challenging in the airport, running around with Daisy. We went into Cairns that night and again we lost Seren. We lost her in the swimming pool too. She was told off but I could see she didn't get it, she didn't realise how scary it is for us and how dangerous it could be. I couldn't find her for about five minutes and again was running around like the crazy mum who had lost her child. The diet is about 90% right, so could the 15% be making all this difference? She is always losing her shoes, her books, her hats – you name it!

5 October
Had a fantastic day! We snorkelled in the Great Barrier Reef and Seren was so brave going off with Daddy and then Mummy (she was braver than me). Everything was going great and then Seren got upset and ran off, eventually coming back.

She has been writing stories and reading them back to us and I have managed to do some poetry with her too, which was lots of fun. I feel she is very creative, so I want to try and help her with this, maybe if I channel her into something it will help?

She seems to get very upset by the smallest thing, and I can't seem to bring her back around. She answers back all the time, she screams at us, runs off, is defiant and she hurts her brother and sister all the time, which makes us so mad!

We have tried everything, we have taken out dairy and gluten, added supplements and meat, homoeopathic treatments, herbs, you name it, and she is worse than ever!

I am now at breaking point. We literally cannot cope anymore as a family. I have made an appointment today to see another pediatrician when we get back.

I'm going to try the reward tomorrow; it's all I've got left as I am at the point now where I just want to beat her, which I would never do, but that's honestly how I feel!

It's having an impact on Daisy too, as her behaviour is starting to change. : -(We have tried everything. We are so lost and confused by it all. I must get some more supplements tomorrow, but with my hand on my heart, I don't believe it has anything to do with them, I think it's just a bit of a placebo effect.

6 October

Today Seren has been screaming uncontrollably. She's been hitting out at me, hysterical and kicking Karl and me.

I smacked her on her hand and it escalated to the point of hysteria!

I am now going to start the Ritalin as we can't cope as a family anymore. The other two children are seeing this. We have tried every- thing but we can't cope. It is impossible to function as a family with this behaviour.

8 October

Today started off well. Seren was helping, being good and doing as she was told. Sadly this changed very quickly – she refused to wear her shoes, but then refused to carry them. She was running off, being defiant, being cheeky, answering back. She told me today that she hated me and she wanted to punch me in the face! She is unbelievable!

9 October

Snatching, grabbing, screaming, fighting, defiant. It has become so bad now that I've resulted in smacking her (and I hate myself for it). I'm at my wit's end. I feel like I hate her and I can't take it anymore. Ritalin when we get back for our sanity.

16 October
I haven't updated this for a week, but it's a never-ending nightmare and this road trip had now become a road hell! We have landed in Bali and her behaviour has been terrible.

It's causing me to be extremely depressed. I feel like I need anti-depressants. I can't cope with her behaviour any longer. I am so, so depressed. :-(I am struggling to cope. When I get home to Australia, I am going to see about getting some counselling for myself, as I really, really can't cope anymore. :-(

17 October
Seren has been at the kids club all day, but as soon as she is back she is defiant, naughty, running off and ignoring us.

Grabbing, pushing, shouting, rude – she is horrible and very, very hard to be around. I literally can't cope anymore.

18–20 October
Seren is now more defiant than ever. She runs off constantly, shouts, is rude, won't do as she is told, she won't follow instructions and is mean to her sister.

She tells me to shut up. She screams at me that she hates me, she calls me a weirdo, it's worse than ever!

Positives are that she is so brave, snorkelling in the Great Barrier Reef, swimming in the ocean. She will try anything and do anything, the more exciting the better. The downsides are that she has no fear and puts herself in danger. She is also so very difficult to control.

I didn't update my diary again for another month. I was depressed, so sad and I felt so helpless. Every day was pretty much the same – Seren was defiant, Seren would run off, Seren would be mean to her brother and sister and scream obscenities at me.

Cue the new pediatrician!

It just goes to show the confusion and the struggle that Karl and I were both feeling. After I had read all the information that my friend Olivia sent on Ritalin and ADHD, I was dead set on not medicating. I was convinced that there could be a more natural way of dealing with Seren's ADHD. I had condemned the pediatricians and hoped that the naturopath could help me, could help Seren. But, after trying everything, we just simply couldn't handle one more day, one more hour, one more second of this relentless shit that we were dealing with every single day.

I couldn't wait to get home and see the new pediatrician that our friends had recommended. When I read his testimonials he seemed excellent. He had a more traditional approach that focused on firm parenting, which I liked. I started to wonder whether ADHD was just a disorder of our times – were we allowing kids to take control of us while we tried parenting them in our 'namby-pamby' way? Maybe we did need to be stricter with Seren? Maybe she just needed a short, sharp smack?

On our holiday, I had spanked her twice – once on her hand and once on her leg. It made me feel awful and it sent her into a screaming fit, so I wasn't sure that this would be the way forward. I thought about my childhood and had mixed feelings about whether being smacked had helped me in any way. To be honest, my thoughts and mind were so clouded that I wasn't sure what I had felt when I was younger, or how I felt anymore.

I called the pediatrician while we were still away and made a date for the end of November. I had heard that he didn't medicate straightaway and that he would help us with our parenting skills – the whole thing excited me and gave me a bit of hope. I started to think of lions in a pack and how you would see the lioness strike her paw at her cubs when they would step out of line. If it worked for the lioness, then surely it would work for me? You don't see the lions talk about their feelings, or put the little cub on the time-out rock – no, they give them a short, sharp smack to put them back on track. Maybe that's what my naughty little cub needed? Perhaps I needed to be more like the lioness in the wild and give Seren a short, sharp strike to get her back in line!

Chapter Five

When the natural alternatives just aren't cutting it (Now where is that pediatrician again?)

I sometimes wonder what it would have been like 100 years ago, or even 1,000 years ago, when we could heal ourselves with a bit of tree sap and some leaves and berries. Unless you are living in a tribe in the wilderness, all of the knowledge that we had as humans has died, and we are all now at the mercy of the doctor's prescription pad!

Diane was Seren's teacher; she was fantastic and we would exchange emails throughout the week about Seren's behaviour. Diane would request a meeting usually once a week so we could work out how best to teach and help Seren. I will be eternally grateful to Diane for spending the time trying to help me during those dark days with Seren.

Correspondence during this time

27 October

Hi Diane,

Being back is good! Seren wrote a travel journal while we were away, so she will bring it to school this week when I've printed the pictures for her. I meant to email you all day, so apologies that you are getting this late. Seren will be off school in the morning but back for lunch (which I believe is 12.30 pm).

We've had a terrible time with Seren while we were away. I feel very sad, as we've tried so hard with her diet, supplements and homoeopathy. It seemed to be working but unfortunately it's now not working at all, and we are finding it increasingly hard to parent her.

I managed to get an appointment with the pediatrician tomorrow morning at 9.45 am. We feel that it's time to look at medication. Seren will also be continuing with the play therapist appointments for another five weeks.

Love Susy xx

28 October

Hi Diane,

So sorry to hear you are not well. I hope you feel better soon.

We saw a fantastic pediatrician today and he's given us some great stuff to help manage Seren's behavior. We are going back to see him in three weeks, so I will keep you posted.

Love Susy xx

29 October

Thanks Susy! I'm getting better.

Let us know when you begin the trial ... she was very calm today.

Diane xx

Appointment with the new pediatrician

When we went to our appointment, Seren seemed scared and cowered on my knee, refusing to look at the pediatrician. I had never seen her like this before with anyone else other than Karl and me. She seemed so frightened, yet part of me did think she was also pretending.

The pediatrician asked us to ignore her behaviour and to continue. We asked if Seren should leave the room and he said that it was fine for her to stay. He felt that Seren needed to understand what was going on.

Given what has happened to Seren and us over the last eighteen months since this appointment, I would now completely disagree with this suggestion. Even if children pretend to play with toys in the corner of the room, or draw a picture or watch television, they are listening to every word you are saying and they are absorbing those words like a sponge!

Difficult, challenging children actually realise that they are difficult and challenging, and they have a very low opinion of themselves and how others view them. During this time, Seren was convinced that no-one liked her. She felt we didn't love her, and that her teachers and her friends didn't like her. She would tell us frequently how she had overheard us talking about her bad behaviour.

I've learnt that children like Seren don't then think, 'Oh no, Mum is upset with me and doesn't like how I am acting, tomorrow I am going to wake up and be really good'. They don't think like that. They build a massive great big wall to protect themselves and it's called 'defiance'. And the more you shout, the more you tell them off, the more you put them in time-out, and the more you openly talk about them with experts, or to partners, the bigger and bigger that wall gets.

And believe me, at the time, trying to be calmer and more loving with my defiant ADHD child was not for the faint-hearted, and I was certainly not in the right state of mind to start doing that. However, in time, I would become a master at it, and Seren's behaviour would go on to have a complete turnaround. Only then would I realise how right the calm and loving approach was for ADHD and defiant kids!

Back to that meeting though ... The pediatrician asked questions all about Seren, her behaviour, her routine, her schooling; he even asked questions about our marriage and our childhoods and I found him very honest and very thorough. He was very kind to us and told us that we were good parents. He said he felt that I was a good mum and that I was trying my best. He did feel that we were too soft with Seren, and that we were inconsistent and needed to be firmer with her. The pediatrician gave us a list of rules and some very thorough guidelines, along with advice on how to implement the new regulations into our household. He was very concise and covered many areas such as emotions of the child and parents. We felt excited that we now had something else to use and it didn't involve medication!

At times, I did struggle to understand the medical terms he used, but overall I liked what he had to say and I was determined to get home and start this new time-out method immediately!

The pediatrician also told us how to manage Seren running off and not coming back. He said we had to decide on a word that we would always use when Seren ran off. She would then serve a time-out as soon as we got home.

This worked incredibly well and still does to this day; this was actually one of the best tools that I had ever come across for bringing Seren back when she ran off. It was a lifesaver! However, it's important to mention, that at the end of this journey, we found that a better way to manage her was to stop time-out altogether. She is now only sent to her room to give herself time to 'calm down'. It is now seen as a positive thing where we give her (and us) some breathing space, as opposed to a negative form of punishment.

More help from Ruth

As I previously mentioned, one of the friends who helped me during this time was my neighbour and landlady in the UK. We had rented Ruth's house for almost four years back in the UK. Ruth would often pop over for coffee and chats, and we promised that we would keep this up when we moved. What started out as friendly emails soon became an online counselling service from Ruth (although I am not sure that she signed up for that)!

Correspondence during this time

10 November

Hi Ruth,

How are you both?
Little Flynn is adorable and he just started walking last week, which was so cute! He is still (thankfully) very chilled! He's so like Daisy, calm and easy! Daisy is doing great at school.

We are having a bit of a tough time with Seren though, but we are trying our best to work through it. We have been seeing a child psychologist to help us with certain things, as Seren is so defiant it was getting hard to manage. The school also picked up very early on her hyperactivity as well as an inability to concentrate, which we totally agree with.

We have also started seeing a great pediatrician who it very old school and believes in being strict with children (especially oppositional and defiant children), which Seren is. She has been diagnosed with ADHD by the psychologist and a different pediatrician, but I have yet to hear what this pediatrician feels. We are seeing him again in another week. We have changed her diet, we all now eat meat, and Seren doesn't eat gluten or dairy and we have seen an improvement in her behaviour. We have a time-out method that we use, and have also tried homoeopathy, herbs and supplements. We have been going down this route since about May, and in some ways it was getting better, but in others there is no improvement. I'm really sad about it, but it does make sense to us, and I am convinced that she has ADHD.

I am starting to look at private schools for the children for high school and there are some amazing ones here in Perth. I am so worried that Seren won't manage with this as she is behind in her reading and she isn't great at making friends due to her impulsively etc. Her friends find her lots of fun in the playground as she has boundless energy, but she is struggling to make friends in the classroom, as her behaviour can be quite disruptive.

I have observed her in the classroom and it was like watching 'Tigger' bounce around the room! She has a fabulous teacher who is working closely with us to help her, and right now the Montessori method is the best for her. I hope we can find the light at the end of the tunnel, I really do. She has such a wonderful side to her; she can be loving and caring and so polite and sweet, but the other side is so hard to cope with! On a positive note, she is doing amazing at swimming and gymnastics and has just started surf club (the positive of ADHD – no fear)! I have begun going to yoga in the park with her on a Saturday to see if it helps to calm her down too.

I said to Karl last night that it's so consuming! I need to be careful that Flynn and Daisy aren't left out in any way as they are so good and don't deserve to be left out. Have you had any experience with this or do you know anyone that has?

What would you do, Ruth? What do you think is the best thing? I have even thought about boarding school, as I know your children went to boarding school, but if she is struggling in Montessori (and they believe she is very bright), then is she going to struggle even more in this environment?

We are growing vegetables and it's so easy as we have so much sun! We are growing herbs, spinach and lettuce. We also have tomatoes and carrots at the moment, oh and we've just bought a lemon tree so we are going to plant that too! The life here is amazing; it's such a beautiful life for the children. We were part of a street festival yesterday and it was so much fun. We were doing a parade with the school, and after that we went for dinner at this beautiful restaurant on the beach – the kids were running around in the sand and the ocean. We watched a beautiful sunset and then we went home and got the children into bed. So beautiful. :-)

Lots of love, Susy xx

PS. The road trip was amazing!! Very hard with an ADHD child (don't know what we were thinking) but we did make lots of memories, and Bali was awesome. Karl had a fabulous 40th!

PPS. I think of you lots, and the lovely house of yours that we lived in – Seren often talks about her room and watching the horses in the fields. Sorry I don't manage to email you as much as I would like, but you are both always in my thoughts.

Dear Susy,

So lovely to hear from you. Looking forward to seeing the photos of the house but I am sure it will be beautiful as you are the best homemaker I know. Glad to hear that Karl is slowly getting his business going. As much as he would like to be a surfer boy, it would probably get him down in the end.

Really sorry to hear about Seren and I was so glad that you gave me all the details and the ways you are trying so hard to avoid the Ritalin, but as you say it is so hard. I did worry that Seren had ADHD before you left, but I thought that it was possible that a complete change of environment and lots of outdoor activity may help the situation. You asked me what my thoughts were, but all I can say is that even though you are trying everything, you may have to succumb to some form of medication in the end.

My daughter's friend has a son with a similar problem. As he grew into a teenager, he only had to take his medication when he had exams, and more regularly to help him do his homework. He is now at Exeter Uni and only resorts to it when he feels it is necessary. I know this is looking ahead but it may be of some comfort. Have you tried getting Seren to play a musical instrument? Another friend's grandson has ADHD and he started the piano and two years later he has won a music scholarship to a good school and is much calmer in his behaviour.

I do not think a boarding school would work for you as a family, or for Seren. She is far too young and she needs you all.

Also, have you joined a help group for parents with the same problem? So lovely to hear that Daisy and Flynn are thriving and they must give you endless joy.

You did mention once that you may come back in the summer. We are away from the 17 July in Italy, so hope it is before then.

Thinking about you all and am keeping up with your Facebook news.

Lots of Love, Ruth

It was never the whole truth

One of the things that I noticed in my email to Ruth is that even though I was baring my soul and telling her of things that were happening with Seren, I was still not telling her the whole truth.

Every day, and I mean every day, was a struggle with Seren. There wasn't a day where we did something or went somewhere with Seren and just had fun! Medication worked for a while, which I will get to shortly, but with that came huge side effects and for me the side effects outweighed the positives every time.

Nothing in life is that simple. I know of someone who has terrible epilepsy and needs medication to control the epilepsy. She is hugely grateful for this medication but it comes at a price, she struggles with her weight and has terrible problems with anxiety and depression brought on by the medication. I wholeheartedly believe in the concept that you can't have your cake and eat it. We can't just be given a pill and suddenly everything is perfect, it's simply not that easy.

In my email to Ruth, I told her about the street festival, dinner on the beach, the kids playing in the sand, and how we had watched the beautiful sunset together. I even posted a picture on Facebook and the kids seemed so happy and smiley, but the real truth was that again it was a day from hell.

Learned behaviour

Seren's school was doing a parade in a local street festival; everyone was so excited about it, everyone except for Seren.

Daisy was doing it too and was dressed up like a little bumble bee.

Everyone smiled and laughed and thoroughly enjoyed it. The drums, the singing, the atmosphere, there was such excitement throughout the streets with people cheering and clapping.

Seren refused to wear her costume and refused to do the parade with all her classmates, so she ended up walking with Daisy's class and us, refusing to smile and hating every second of it. Afterwards, we went for dinner to a cafe near the beach. It overlooked the ocean and all the children were playing in the park outside. It was a kid haven – full of happy, smiling, excitable children, and then there was Seren. She was so sad, so full of anger, so difficult!

She refused to get out of the car, as she wasn't happy with what she was wearing. We finally got her out of the car and into the cafe, but then she ran straight out, curled up in a ball and started rocking herself. She reminded me of a bear I once saw at the Perth Zoo. It paced up and down and seemed so agitated, upset and bored! The enclosure looked quite small, and I found myself questioning the zoo, but then I noticed a sign on the window. It told us how the bear had been rescued from poachers, and as a cub it had been beaten, abused, starved and chained up for most of the day. He now resided in the zoo with a beautiful, happy environment where they even played games with him to keep his brain occupied. But the pacing was 'learned behaviour' from such a young age, and he was unable to stop doing it. They had taken him away from the horrible environment, but even with love, activities, and care, he couldn't stop walking back and forth.

Watching the bear made me realise that I had to change Seren's environment. We had to learn how to parent her, as whatever we were doing was clearly not working! All the other parents that day were looking at us. I could tell they were judging us, and I don't blame them.

Just like I judged the zoo that day, I knew that these other parents could be doing the same to us. Maybe they thought that we were cruel, evil parents who apparently beat up their child, because every time we walked up to Seren she screamed like we were going to hurt her and then she would run off crying and frightened.

Honestly, as a parent, it was crushing and utterly heartbreaking. I didn't know what to do when she acted that way. I never saw other children running away from their parents, screaming and crying. *Is it just us? Why is this happening? What were we doing wrong?* Just like the zoo, I wished we could have walked around with a little sign. If we could all write a sign about our child, would it stop people judging, commenting, assuming? Would it make us assess our parenting if we did have a sign?

'Our daughter has ADHD and ODD. She is under the care of both a psychologist and pediatrician and soon we will be medicating her, so hopefully her behaviour will be better. Please bear (excuse the pun here) with us, thank you.'

ADHD in the olden days

I once read an example of ADHD in the olden days. In my dad's youth, kids would run around the back streets with dirty faces, playing in alleyways with conkers, and there was no such thing as ADHD. Little Jonny would always be difficult for his mother to handle, he would run amok, and everyone in the neighbourhood knew who he was. His mother would give him a clip around the ear and send him off outside, and then all the neighbours would keep an eye on him, making sure he didn't get into trouble and giving his mother a well-deserved break before he came back at dusk.

Childhood isn't like that anymore; it's a lot more full-on for parents, especially mothers who can't send their kids out to run amok anymore, giving themselves a few hours peace. We can barely let them out of our sight. *Is that the reason that children are becoming more anxious?* Even in my childhood, I was off from a young age, running, climbing, bike riding, making tree houses, dens, having conker fights and playing hopscotch and skipping games.

These activities have been replaced with Netflix, iPads, Xboxes, hyperactivity-inducing preservatives, additives, and hormone-changing herbicides and pesticides. And while these activities can't be blamed solely for the rise in ADHD, I think they need to take some responsibility. Then there is the added worry about pedophiles and child snatchers. *Are our children simply a by-product of our First World lifestyle?*

Handling the tough moments

The screaming, crying and running away behaviour that Seren displayed was so hard to deal with. And she still does it now, but not as often. Thankfully, I have finally learnt how to handle these moments; it doesn't faze me anymore, I just go with it.

In fact, she did it only today as I was writing this section. We had gone away for the weekend to support our friend who was running in the iron man competition. As Seren can't cope with change, a lot of the older behaviours started again – defiance, running off, screaming and shouting 'don't hurt me'. But now it doesn't bother me. I know not to get angry, not to take it personally. I use positive reinforcement to bring her back around and then very quickly she will apologise and say, 'Mummy, I love you so much, thank you'.

And this is such a huge thing for me, as I feel that I have cracked it (at least for now).

Seren will always be difficult. Simple things, such as pins and needles in her foot, will always end up with Seren screaming like someone is chopping off her leg. A change in breakfast can sometimes make Seren cry and lose the plot; she can't cope with simple, reasonable changes.

But the difference now is that I try not to overthink it, I don't whisk her off to visit the pediatrician or the psychologist. I don't turn to medication to try and make her like everyone else. I accept it, and I love her just a little bit more for who she is. I trust in the process and believe that it will get easier the older she gets. I don't believe in conforming anymore. I give her clear boundaries surrounded by positivity and love.

During the hard times, Karl's mum, Mary, would always say, 'Seren just needs more love'. At the time, we were struggling so much that I found these comments dismissive and unsupportive.

I wanted to know what was wrong with Seren, not faff about trying to be more fluffy and loving. I was on a mission and I had to make things right.

Why was Seren like this? What is wrong? How can we fix her?

But Seren didn't need fixing; just like Mary said, she needed an abundance of love, in fact, she needed a tsunami tidal wave of love! Mary was so right but I wouldn't realise how accurate her love comments were until the very end of the journey. While there were many things that we needed to change, love was one that we definitely needed to express more with Seren!

Seren is Seren. She is ADHD, and she will always struggle with these things, but I have learnt how to parent her without medication. And hopefully, I am giving her the tools and strategies that, over time, will be so ingrained into her psyche that she will grow and shine, and she will not need medication to function or to survive.

We managed to bring Seren round that day, but she refused to come back into the restaurant and sat curled up in a ball outside by the sand dune. After dinner, we all went down to the beach, and Seren ran around having fun, smiling and laughing

But the journey her behaviour took us on every day was so hard, so challenging, and so depressing, that we wondered why we ever bothered doing anything as a family!

Diary entries during this time

18 November
We saw the new pediatrician today again and discussed supplements, behaviour, anxiety, psychologist, school etc. Seren got upset while we were in his office, but overall she was ok. We need to continue with the time-out method.

19 November
Seren has started to become very difficult and is crying a lot when going to bed. She wanted a sleepover with her sister but I told her she couldn't, as she hadn't been good before bedtime – this didn't end well.

She was being very hyper and started having pillow fights with everyone (although no-one else was playing). I am still finding it hard.

20 November
Seren is all over the place. Her routine is out the window; she gets upset about her breakfast, her clothes, and her shoes. We get into the car late – she's screaming. We go swimming after school, all good. We go for fish, and her behaviour is hyper. She is running around, leaving the table, running out of the restaurant. She won't have her special drink. She goes to bed screaming 'get off me'. Screaming, crying, slamming doors, throwing stuff at the door. She screams at me, 'Shut up, Mum. I hate you, leave me alone'.

21 November
Again our routine is all over the place. She's started moving her room around again, all her furniture is being moved. She makes her bed differently. She is changing.
She's running up and down the stairs like a crazy person – it's chaos! Karl told me the psychologist thinks it's my fault and Seren is scared of me, and that's why she is acting this way. I am desperately unhappy and so sad. Must talk to the pediatrician about ADHD, child bipolar and medication?

Psychologist vs. pediatrician

Seren continued her appointments to see the same psychologist on Thursday at 1.00 pm, but as I needed to collect Daisy from school at that time, Karl would take Seren to her appointments.

With so many different appointments to see different people, my head was in a spin. And with two little ones, it was becoming difficult. Karl didn't mind because he felt that it would give him a bit of one-on-one time with Seren.

Seren had been seeing this psychologist for seven months now; she had diagnosed Seren with ADHD, anxiety and low self-esteem. She had also witnessed Seren be diagnosed with ADHD with the first pediatrician and medicated with Ritalin. She had then seen us take Seren off Ritalin, change her diet, use homoeopathy, naturopathy and supplements.

She had witnessed positive changes in Seren. Although she still felt that Seren didn't have a good memory and would continually forget what she was doing during play therapy, she did feel her anxiety was better.

She had encouraged me to praise Seren instantly when she did something good, ignore the bad and to talk to Seren about her emotions, even giving us an 'emotions' handout that we put up on the wall in the kitchen. She encouraged me to discuss anger, sadness, happiness etc. with Seren, so Seren could explain how she was feeling.

When I think back, it was very similar to the film *Inside Out*, which I would recommend parents watch with their child. It's an amazing movie and can help children be more aware of their emotions. I found that, after watching the film with Seren, we would often refer to it and she could clearly talk about her feelings and her moods.

Even though we were doing all of this, and we felt that we had tried everything, Seren's behaviour was still awful. Despite our very best efforts, we would once again need to consider medication to help Seren.

Our family was being torn apart. I was at my wit's end and even though we had spent thousands of dollars, and seen numerous experts, she was still no better. Things seemed to work for a while – when we changed her diet, her behaviour seemed so much better. Then when we tried homoeopathy and naturopathy, her behaviour appeared to improve, even her teacher noticed a difference.

But during the road trip, Seren became so out of control that, despite all our best efforts, we felt we needed more help. We were at a total loss as to how to parent her.

The new pediatrician talked to us at length about how he completely disagreed with psychologists. He felt that we were giving Seren mixed messages. He felt we were too soft with her and that Seren knew how to manipulate us. He said she was very bright. He told us that Seren could see my weakness and knew how to play me, and that talking about emotions would only give her more room to be defiant.

Even though we felt Seren did have ADHD, the biggest problem for us was her defiance. We discussed this issue at length, and the pediatrician referred to this defiance as ODD (Oppositional Defiance Disorder).

Can you imagine how hard it was when Seren couldn't carry out a single instruction?

'Seren, please put your school shoes on?' 'NO.'

'Seren, please make your bed?'

'NO.'

'Seren, please give this drink to Daisy?'

'NO'.

'Seren, please come now, we need to leave for school?' 'NO'.

'Seren, please get out of the car?'

'NO.'

Every request, every question, every plea, would always be answered with, 'NO'. However, most of the time, Seren wouldn't even answer us, she would simply ignore us. This defiance was one of the most important issues we needed to get on top of.

The time-out method

We implemented the recommended time-out method straightaway and started to get instant results from it. We stopped talking about our emotions and how we felt. We also just put up the house rules in the kitchen and if Seren didn't do as she was told, without any chances, she would go on time-out in her bedroom.

We always found this hard and it's not as if Seren would say, 'Sure, sorry about that Mummy, I will head up to my bedroom now'. Seren would be protesting, screaming and fighting with us. We would have to carry her screaming and shouting as we took her upstairs. It got so bad that it was impossible to get her upstairs sometimes. Not only that, it made us desperately sad as our little girl screamed, kicked and fought with us as we tried to put her in her room. Seren was quite tall for her age, so carrying a tall, heavy seven-year-old into her room was becoming impossible for me. We eventually agreed that the time-out room would be the laundry room, at least then it wasn't too far for us to carry Seren.

Seren would be on time-out anywhere from five to sometimes ten times a day. It was so hard as she would protest, scream, shout, rant and rave at us. She would kick and punch the laundry door and throw things at it. It was not only hard to witness Seren's behaviour, but also to know that Daisy and Flynn had to witness it all as well. This would upset me greatly.

Most of the time I would stay calm and even though she was kicking the living daylights out of the door, I would say nothing and just let her serve her time-out. I would often have to hold the handle as she would protest and try and open the door.

After every appointment with the pediatrician, he would ask to see us in a month's time. However, Seren's behaviour would be so bad that after only two weeks, I would call his office and plead with the receptionist for an appointment that day. She was so lovely and would always try and squeeze me in that day or the next day.

I would arrive calm, composed and well dressed with my diary and notepad in hand. I would explain in detail how Seren's behaviour was worse than ever and ask what we could do about the situation and how could he help me. It was a horrible feeling, baring my soul to the pediatrician and sharing my innermost fears and concerns about my child. He was very kind and would always reassure me that I was doing a great job, that I was a great mum and that it would get better.

I really liked him and would look forward to our meetings. In those dark times, he was all I had. I had complete and utter faith in him and I would do anything that he suggested. With his particular time-out method, he reminded me that we shouldn't shout, raise our voice, get angry or emotional, we had to stay calm. This was so hard when Seren was beating the door down.

He said that very quickly she would realise who was boss, and she'd understand that I wouldn't be controlled or manipulated. He went on to explain that this method wouldn't make a change overnight and that it would take time before we saw any improvement. And unfortunately it could often get worse before it got better.

Dumping the psychologist?

Our new pediatrician also felt very strongly that we had two choices and two choices only. We were to either use his time-out method, or use the psychologist's method (which was to talk about emotions). He felt that we absolutely could not use a combination of the two. He felt we were wasting our money, as the two methods clashed.

I took on board what he had said, but Seren loved her weekly visits with the psychologist, and Seren's teacher also praised the psychologist for helping Seren with her friendships. She felt that Seren's behaviour in school was better, she was making friends, and this was all down to the psychologist. Diane only had great things to say about her, so it didn't feel like the right time to say goodbye.

Psychologist vs. pediatrician vs. naturopath

The psychologist had repeatedly told me that I should implement one thing at a time, so we could see what was working.

However, the naturopath felt very differently and said that we needed to change lots of things in Seren's routine straightaway. She felt that we should eliminate gluten and dairy immediately from Seren's diet, adding fish oils, supplements, homoeopathy and herbs, as they would work together in harmony to help Seren with her ADHD.

The psychologist strongly disagreed with this advice and told me that I was inconsistently moving from one thing to the other, not knowing what was working and not working.

And looking back, maybe I was chopping and changing everything and maybe I did prolong things or make matters worse. However, at the time I was given so much conflicting advice, it was hard to know who was right.

But having gone through it, I now feel that the naturopath was 100% right! I would personally recommend that you have your child tested for everything, either through a doctor or a naturopath, and whatever they are deficient in, get that into your child!

I would also suggest you add a good fish oil, a probiotic, zinc and magnesium (at night, as this helps them to sleep). I would also recommend using essential oils for calming, grounding and concentration.

And clean their diet up as much as possible. We always choose savoury over sweet for Seren and take gluten and dairy out as much as we can, although we relax this slightly at the weekends. Look out for changes with certain foods, noting them in your diary, and use chemical-free products on them. Become a master at looking at food labels; it will shock you when you realise what is really in food! A great book to help you is The Chemical Maze, by Bill Statham. It explains exactly what is in your food and what effect it can have on your children.

The psychologist also disagreed with us taking Seren off medication and made it very clear that she didn't agree with the different things that we were trying. As Karl was taking Seren to see the psychologist every Thursday, she would say these things to Karl and then he would pass on all of her comments to me. It would upset me that she couldn't realise that I was only trying my best.

I asked Karl to explain to her that I was documenting everything in a diary and that I was consistent. There was a plan, but maybe it didn't seem like that to other people. All I knew was that I had to be sure that I had tried everything and anything before we medicated Seren again. I had to know that I had given my daughter a chance.

One thing for me to remember is that all the experts were just trying to advise me in the best way that they could. They were masters in their fields, having studied long and hard, dedicating their lives to helping children. I am not against them or their methods, and I am truly grateful for their help with Seren. Everyone was just trying their best for my family and me.

A naturopath opts for natural methods and treats the child holistically.

The psychologist will assess and deal with the child's emotional, behavioural and developmental difficulties, and help find positive ways for parents to interact with them.

The pediatrician is a medical doctor with specialised training and skills in the diseases and illnesses that affect the health and development of babies, children and teenagers. Pediatricians know a lot about the many different conditions and illnesses that can affect children's health, welfare, behaviour and education, but fundamentally their 'go-to' method is medication.

Each specialist has a method, a plan, a formula of dealing with an ADHD child. For many parents, the naturopath may be enough, and changing their child's diet and adding supplements can often work. For others, a change in parenting and regular visits to the psychologist can have a positive effect on the child, but for most, the medication given by the pediatrician is often the route that many parents choose.

Seren was becoming worse

Seren was starting to act very strangely and her behaviour was becoming more and more alarming. She had begun to have anxiety attacks, which after a while we realised were panic attacks, but at the time I didn't even know that this could happen to a child. Can a child of seven, who came from a loving, happy home, have panic attacks?

Diary entries during this time

28 November
We are excited today because Seren has been invited to a party. I took her out for the day to buy her a new dress. The day was spent in the pool, watching a movie and doing craft. Mummy takes her to the party; she's great.

After thirty minutes I saw her walk off from her friends and go to the trampoline. She hurt her knee and started crying. She then spent the next two hours sitting on the same chair. She didn't join in with the dancing and singing and didn't eat anything. She seemed very sad, didn't play with her friends, and then we went home.

When we got home she told me that she hates parties. She doesn't like being in crowds and doesn't like dancing as she is worried what people will say about her. She went to bed crying. :-(She also stated that she didn't play at the party as she hurt her leg.

30 November
Seren woke up crying, her leg was hurting and she said she couldn't go to school. She ran off back to bed. I went up with a coffee and a hot chocolate and we talked about our emotions etc. I told her she could wear something lovely and I'll do something nice with her hair. I managed to bring her around and she went to school. She didn't go to gymnastics again; she said she has an injury.

2 December
Seren came down in her dressing gown this morning. She didn't want breakfast and wouldn't get dressed. She went into time-out after we tried other different methods to try and bring her around – talking about our feelings and failed negotiations. She screamed and started battering the doors. She then went back on time-out.

This continued until about ten minutes of kicking, screaming etc. I tried to remain calm and look after the other two children. Jenny, the babysitter, arrived as she was looking after Flynn today for me this morning. A couple of tradesman arrived at 8.00 am and had a chat with Karl about some electricity jobs.

After Seren's time-out finished, she ran upstairs and took off all her clothes and then hid under her bed. I reverted back to talking about our emotions, as the time-out is definitely not working!

I managed to get her dressed (forty-five minutes later), she calmed down but started saying she's scared of me, then she's scared of Karl, and she's also scared of the imaginary spider again (this happens a lot). She then ran out of the house, screaming, spitting, hands and feet clawed. This is ridiculous; we couldn't get her to school. Karl took Daisy to school and Seren stayed with me, but I was so cross with her that I sent her to her room. Ten minutes later she was fine.

The spider web or devil-possessed child?

I remember another time when Seren got a spider web stuck on her finger (as I mentioned in my diary). She had been playing in the pool when she got out, as she wanted to dive back in. She climbed out of the pool and accidentally brushed past one of our bushes that we have near the pool, getting the finest bit of cobweb on her finger. When she noticed it, she let out the biggest scream. It was a scream that was panic, it was fear, it was deafening, and again I was so worried what the neighbours would think!

I was in the kitchen and Daisy and Flynn were hanging around the pool with Karl. I could see that he was sick of this happening, so he ignored her and just let her get on with it.

Around this time, Seren was having regular random panic attacks, like this spider episode, sometimes twice a day. They would be about anything, but mostly they were directed at Karl and me. When I look back now, I realise that these anxiety episodes only started after we implemented the new time-out method. However, the time-out method did seem to be working for us, so we didn't link the two (hindsight is such a great thing!).

That day, Seren was frozen in fear, screaming, wide-eyed with her fingers and feet clawed and hyperventilating. Karl was still ignoring her and even though I was sick of it as well, and wasn't sure if she was pretending, I couldn't just sit back and not help her. I went over to Seren, but she was now scared of me too. Her eyes were wild and she looked at me like I was a monster, like I would hurt her in some way. I was her mummy. I only wanted to love her and help her – it was so hard. I wrapped a towel around her and tried to calm her down, but it took over fifteen minutes to stop her from screaming and crying like she had just been involved in a shark attack. As she always did, she eventually stopped crying and then moved on, jumping into the pool to continue playing, totally unfazed by what had happened.

I always felt that she would create this crazy, screaming drama and then be happy again, yet everyone around her was completely shaken up about what had happened.

Later that day, Seren let Daisy into the pool area, even though she had been told repeatedly not to do this as Daisy couldn't swim and could drown. Seren would drag a chair to the pool fence, stand on it, reach over and open the gate, letting her sister in. Even though Seren was an excellent swimmer, we had told her repeatedly not to do this. She was to always ask us first and she must always have an adult watching her. To take her sister in the pool was so irresponsible.

Karl was so cross with Seren as he felt that, at age seven, Seren should have some responsibility and shouldn't keep letting Daisy into the pool. As punishment, Karl told Seren to get out of the pool immediately, and she was not allowed to get back into the pool again that day. He explained that her sister could have drowned! Seren started to have one of her fits again – wide-eyed, spitting, drooling, clawed fingers and toes. It was moments like this that we felt that maybe, after all, she was making these episodes up; however, they were pretty convincing!

Again I calmed her down and all was well in our household.

At bedtime, Seren wanted Daddy to read her a book and he said he wouldn't as she had been told off that day for letting her sister go into the pool. He explained that if she was a good girl, she could have a book tomorrow night.

This is when the drama of all dramas started, which would see me Googling 'child devil possession'. *I wonder whether this has happened to other people?*

Seren started to have one of her attacks again. This was now the third one since lunchtime, and believe me they were horrendous to witness and be a part of. This attack was particularly bad and Seren was gasping for breath and couldn't breathe. I came up to see what was happening and I was so shocked that I ran downstairs, grabbed a bag and then held it over Seren's mouth to slow down her breathing. She took about three or four minutes to calm down and then proceeded to fall asleep on my lap with me stroking her head. She seemed to be asleep so I lifted her up and lay her in bed, still stroking her head and her soft blonde hair. Tears ran down my face as I looked at Karl and whispered to him, 'What is wrong with our daughter? What is happening? I am so scared Karl.'

Seren was lying on her bed, eyes closed, with the blankets over her and the lights down low. It was a calm, serene moment, but then Seren started to smile and this freaked both of us out because we thought she was asleep. *Why would a sleeping child be smiling as her parents sat on her bed unhappy, confused and quietly crying?*

It haunted Karl and me, and at that moment we were worried that something was very wrong with Seren. I was so scared that I left the room and went downstairs and cried. Karl joined me moments later. 'Karl, what is wrong with Seren? I am starting to think that she is possessed by the devil!'

I know how silly that seems, what a ridiculous thing to say about your child, but all was not right at all.

I did Google 'child possession' and as Seren wasn't climbing the wall, talking in devil tongue and contorting her body, I suddenly felt so stupid to think that she could have been possessed. But at least I could cross it off the list – phew, thank God for that!

Weeks later, Seren told us that she had pretended to be asleep that night, as she wanted to hear what we would say about her. She said she started to smile because she got embarrassed that she was pretending to be asleep. *Remember what I said about children listening?* Children get it! Children can feel that they are not liked, not loved. And feeling not loved, particularly as a child, is one of the worst things that you can feel. With this feeling comes rejection, then rebellion. I know this, as this is exactly what I felt and what I did when I was a teenager.

Another medication?

The very next day I called the helpful receptionist at the pediatrician's office. After she heard my desperate voice again, she squeezed me in on the Monday for an urgent appointment.

It was 7th December, and we had been seeing the new pediatrician for six weeks, implementing everything that he had said. I was also still giving Seren supplements and fish oils, but things were getting worse, much worse. I was now starting to believe that maybe Seren did need medication.

I went to see the pediatrician but this time I was alone. I told him all about the weekend and what had happened with Seren, and he prescribed her Prozac. He felt that despite our efforts with the time-out method, she was suffering from anxiety and panic attacks, and the Prozac would help.

I told him about my fears about Seren taking medication and his reply was that Prozac was one of the safest drugs on the market. He also mentioned that it was very successful in treating adults and children who were suffering from anxiety and or depression.

It felt wrong to be giving a seven-year-old child an antidepressant. I had always believed that depression and anxiety didn't start until much later in life, and I am still not sure that I believe you are born with a mental illness.

Seren's behaviour twelve months ago was so bad that we thought she was bipolar or had schizophrenia. She screamed so loud that it was as though she was possessed. It was so frightening and haunting to witness as a parent; we were convinced that something was very, very wrong. But Prozac? I guess it was time to try it ...

Now panic attacks ...

At the time of going to see the pediatrician, Seren was having panic attacks up to three times per day. Within days of taking the Prozac, these panic attacks changed to just one per week. Her attacks were still hard and draining, and they were very upsetting for Karl and me to witness, but at least they were only happening now once a week. This was so much easier for us to cope with as a family.

Here is an email that I sent to the pediatrician five weeks after medicating Seren with Prozac.

> Seren has been taking the Prozac medication for the last five weeks and we have seen an overall improvement in the anxiety/panic attacks that she had every day, sometimes twice a day. We only have one of these episodes now each week, but it's interesting that they now only develop when Seren can't have her way.
>
> We are continuing with the time-out method and Seren can be on time-out anywhere from twice to ten times per day. We notice that when there is a change in routine, it can really affect her and she spends most of the day being defiant.

The other thing that is alarming me is that Seren frequently talks of death. It has calmed down now; however, when my parents and brother and his partner arrived three weeks ago, she talked a lot about jumping off a bridge and she talked frequently about what is would be like to die. I really do feel though that she does this as a shock factor. Karl sat her down and talked to her about this and she explained that she says it to be funny or silly. She seems to say a lot of things lately as if to upset people, especially me, but I am continuing to be really calm and not let her see that it is worrying me. She seems beyond her years and yet she doesn't have access to computer games, TV etc. The children may sit down to watch a film most days but these are all innocent, so I am so confused as to where she has learnt this behaviour?

Seren can also hurt her sister Daisy a lot too. She plays very rough and is vindictive and mean to Daisy. This almost goes beyond sibling rivalry, and this behaviour has been noted by all family members since Daisy was born. She talks frequently about the fact that she is not part of this family, no-one loves her, and that she will escape and leave and go to another family.

A lot of the time we find her sneaking behind doors listening to conversations. Another thing is that at times I have described her episodes as being possessed. I know this seems silly but sometimes it's the only way I can describe it. What's scared me is that my dad also felt this, even though I have never said to him that I have felt this way too. Seren's behaviour has really unnerved us all over the last few weeks.

At times Seren is charming, polite, courteous and kind, and other times she is vindictive, spiteful and manipulative. I found her yesterday with her hands underneath the electric garage doors as they were closing, only inches away from her hands. She said she wanted to know what it felt like. We have also found her climbing the gates in our house, which have very large spikes on the end! She has also been stealing money, make up, anything she can get her hands on!

What's so upsetting is that her younger sister and brother are witnessing all this and it's worrying me what affect this is having on them. I absolutely adore my children and I am at a complete loss as to, firstly, what is wrong with Seren and, secondly, what we can do about it. Do you think that she needs to be assessed by a psychiatrist as well as seeing you? I am even at times considering boarding school, but again I am unsure whether this would be the right choice.

Kind regards, Susy

What to say? What to do?

As I read back on this email, I want to burst out crying as I honestly can't believe that I felt like that about my daughter. I want to be transported back in time so I can hug her so tight that I never let her go. I want to tell her how much I love her, and that she is the most beautiful thing that I have seen. I want to protect her and hold her and stop throwing her out to the wolves. I want to take her away and spend the weekend laughing and hugging and holding hands, but we all know that the past is the past.

When I think back on the things that I have said to Seren, I cringe. We have all done it, we have all said things that we regret, but when you have a difficult child it's so much easier to say unkind things, as they push you to almost insanity.

'Why are you so difficult?'

'Why do you have to be so naughty?'

'Why can't you just do as you are told?'

'Why can't you just be good like Daisy?'

I am sure that I probably once told her that I hated her. A friend said to me once that ADHD kids are hard to love and I was able to relate to her so much, in fact it made complete sense! It must have been so hard for Seren to witness, as Daisy was so easy to love. We couldn't understand how we had two entirely different children. *How can you parent them the same, love them the same and yet they can both be so different?* However, if I am honest, we didn't parent them the same.

Imagine being told, or not even being told but feeling that there is something wrong with you, that you are a bad person or you were born naughty. These are all the things that Seren said to us on a daily basis:

'I was born naughty.'

'I am different to everyone else.'

'I am not part of this family.'

'My brain works differently.'

'You hate me.'

'I hate you.'

'I wish I had never been born.'

And the most disturbing comments only started when she began taking Prozac:

'I wonder what it's like to die.'

'I wish I was dead.'

'I wonder what it would be like if I died; would I be on the front cover of those magazines? Would I be famous?'

'I wonder what would happen if I jumped over that bridge and died.'

'Would you be sad if I died?'

'My brain tells me to be bad.'

'I can't stop these bad thoughts in my brain.'

You tell your pediatrician that your daughter has made these comments, and *BOOM*, you are on the road to antipsychotics right there! It's like a prescription is already being written even before you have walked into any pediatrician's office! And when you tell them you keep a diary and this only started a week after your child started taking medication, they insist, 'Oh, it has got nothing to do with that', or, 'She is doing it because she wants the attention'.

I am not here to disparage the experts, believe me I am not. However, what I will do is be brutally honest and then people can make their own minds up.

The pediatrician had complete faith in his medicine, but all my instincts told me otherwise.

It is down to us as parents to do what we feel is the right thing for our children; we know them better than anyone else. Watch, observe, document, review – look at this as a project at work. Try and take out the worry, the emotion, and systematically work through the issues, like your life depended on it.

Karen and I went to see the pediatrician. He had highlighted some points in the email that I had sent him, and asked me questions like: 'Does Seren hurt animals?' 'Is Seren obsessed with fire?' 'Does Seren refuse to obey adults or teachers?' 'Does Seren have an obsession with knives?' 'Does Seren lie?'

This was a very scary conversation, and I couldn't believe that I was having this type of conversation about my beautiful daughter. What the hell has happened to her and why is she acting this way?

We talked with the pediatrician for an hour. We discussed stimulant drugs and he felt they would cause the defiance to become worse. We discussed epilepsy drugs but he felt they would take too long to take effect, and as Seren's behaviour was becoming dangerous we needed to do something that would take effect quickly.

Someone is going to get hurt!

As I wrote in my email, I found Seren with her hands under the electric gate the day after she sliced Daisy's fingernail off. She told me that she felt so awful about hurting Daisy that she wanted to see what it felt like if she hurt her hands too. On the same day, she showed her brother and sister how to climb through the railings of the gates and escape. It was absolute chaos at our home! She was a danger to herself and also to her brother and sister, who were only three and one at the time.

Life was crazy. We had to do something, and as my parents said, 'Someone is going to get hurt or, even worse, have a serious accident'.

It honestly felt like our lives were completely and utterly out of control.

We would still enjoy days out, dinner dates and barbecues, but we were starting to become very isolated, as we often wouldn't want to go out with friends. We had only been living in Australia for a year and I just couldn't bear to meet up with new friends as they would very quickly see that there was a huge problem with Seren.

Oppositional Defiance Disorder too?

The pediatrician was still hesitant to diagnose Seren, but he said that looking at all the evidence and her behaviour, he felt that she had ADHD and ODD (Oppositional Defiance Disorder).

He asked us what was most problematic for us, and without a shadow of a doubt we said the defiance. Yes, Seren was hyperactive, impulsive, and her behaviour was out of control, but the defiance was like a scary, big, stubborn monster that was more powerful and stronger than all of us, and it could literally destroy your inner being with its power and determination.

We felt we had to do something, and do something quick!

The pediatrician recommended a drug called Risperidone, which he felt would be ideal for Seren as it was a mood stabiliser. He also said that it could make her sleepy and we may have to adjust the dosage.

We left that day, and at this point I didn't know much about the drug but I was about to Google the living daylight out of it as soon as I got home. Again, I went to a different chemist, as I couldn't bear for them to think I was medicating Seren so much. I had a prescription for Ritalin at one chemist, a prescription for Prozac at another chemist, and now a prescription for Risperidone at another!

Little did I know that there would soon be many more prescriptions and I would need to go to many more chemists before the problem was sorted!

Chapter Six

Sometimes you have to lose yourself, to find yourself

When I was a child I used to love playing hide and seek. The excitement of trying to hide from someone was what made the game so much fun. I wish I could have gone back to those times, for someone to find me, rescue me, save me. I was now so lost among the craziness that I had completely forgotten the rules of the game.

My lucky number has always been thirteen, and many years ago I discovered that it was also my dad's favourite number, and my late grandma's too, so it was even more special. My first date with Karl was on the 13th. We found out I was pregnant with Flynn on the 13th. And we moved to Australia on the 13th. The 13th has also brought many other magical moments over the last decade (even if it was unlucky for some).

Risperidone ...

The 13th of January wasn't a good day, as I had to pick up a prescription for antipsychotic medication for my seven-year-old daughter. There are many different types of medication used for ADHD, but as Seren had also been diagnosed with ODD, she was prescribed an antipsychotic called Risperidone. It was originally designed for schizophrenia, then bipolar, and in more recent times, prescribed for children with autism and ODD.

There has been growing concern about the rising use of such drugs among children but whether we feel this is right or wrong, morally acceptable or not, the pediatricians are writing these prescriptions because parents are desperately asking them for help. Parents are at their wit's end, not able to parent the child, and it is destroying their mental health, their family and their lives.

I know this, because this was how we felt.

Like other parents, we didn't want to medicate Seren; however, despite trying everything, we were at the end of the line and had nowhere else to turn. Seren was putting herself and her siblings in danger and we had to do something.

... And Prozac

Seren was still taking 20 mg of Prozac, which I later learnt was probably four times too much (although many experts would deny this). We had seen positives with her anxiety, but the side effects from this drug had developed a 'Darth Vader' dark side to her personality. This darker side wasn't Seren's real character, and shortly after stopping the medication, 'Darth Vader' Seren also vanished.

The dark thoughts, comments about death, strange ways and looks weren't her true personality, they were brought on by the medication. I'm conscious not to make this book an 'anti-medication' book, as I have always felt medication has a place, but I have to be honest. When Seren was prescribed Risperidone, she was still taking Prozac as the pediatrician said the two would work well together. I have to admit the Risperidone did work, but the original recommended dose made her sleep for an entire day.

The first day Seren took the Risperidone, she fell asleep shortly after taking it. We were spending the day at the zoo. She was in such a deep sleep that she was unable to open her eyes for more than a few seconds. We couldn't wake her, so we had to push her around in the double buggy for most of the day. Seren would wake to have a drink or something to eat and then the medication would suck her back into sleep again.

It was such a sad day for Seren and our family, but one of the easiest days that we have ever had at the zoo. There was no running off, being defiant, losing her, shouting at her, countless time-outs. We could all breathe and relax. But at the same time, the feelings of guilt and shame were growing in epic proportions.

I always had such a huge interest in the holistic lifestyle, but through sheer desperation I had arrived here at this point, medicating my seven-year-old daughter with such a potent drug that I had to push her around in a baby buggy. To say I hated myself was an understatement.

Diary entries during this time

14 January
We tried Seren on 0.5 mg the next day and again she slept for most of the day. She seemed very peaceful but so did the household! This has certainly given us all some respite from the nightmare that we have been having lately.

15 January
We gave Seren 0.25 mg, and she was great and there were no time-outs! She washed the dishes for me, brought the washing in, sorted the laundry and put it in the bedrooms. She even helped her brother and sister eat their dinner. Played in the pool with Daisy without trying to drown her and is now playing tea party with her siblings.

Another letter to the pediatrician

20 January
We are coming to see you in a week, but I just wanted to email a video I took of Seren this morning before we arrive on Tuesday.
As you suggested, we tried Seren last week on half a tablet of Risperidone and it still made her very drowsy and she slept for most of the day. We left it a day and then tried her on a quarter. We've had an incredible response and Seren has been fantastic, not receiving any time-outs. I do feel, however, it was also in conjunction with the fact my parents have gone home, so our routine has gone back to normal.
Seren was due to go to a music workshop today, but like most of the extra-curricular activities in her life, she said she didn't want to go anymore. She said that she doesn't like people telling her what to do. I tried to get her to go and she refused, which resulted in her running

away. She got back into the car and hit me! My reaction was to hit her back. I didn't hit her, I accidentally hit the chair, but Seren ran out of the car and ran off.

It ended in this behaviour (as seen on the video) and I wanted your opinion, as I feel that she may need to be assessed by a psychiatrist. I believe Seren can control her behaviour until she comes across a situation where she wants her way, and then this happens. It's unbelievable, and I'm at a total loss as to how to manage this as a parent. Would the quarter be doing anything at all? Should we go back and try half tomorrow? Did you ever hear from the lady you recommended that does the behavioural classes? We would be very keen to start this ASAP.

Kind regards, Susy

The music class

The music class day was horrendous, and it was another clear indication that we were still in crisis management. Seren got out of the car and was running towards the road, so Karl had run after her. He grabbed her and put her in the car and she was screaming so much that people walking by must have thought we had stolen her.

She refused to wear her seatbelt (something that happened a lot) and she screamed and kicked the back of the car. She shouted that she hated us and she demanded that we stop the vehicle. As we were driving along, Seren again opened the car door and jumped out of the car. Karl stopped the car and then grabbed her and put her back in the car. She screamed so loud, 'Let me out, let me out, let me out, let me out of this car now'. She screamed and cried, and even typing this now makes me upset. *How and why is this happening with our seven-year-old daughter?* Her behaviour wasn't getting better – it was getting worse.

Other relationships

Seren's behaviour was taking its toll on our relationship – we were at our wit's end, emotional, scared and so unsure of what to do next. I was so homesick and desperately wanted to go back to the UK. I wanted the support of my friends and my family. I missed them so much and I felt like we were drowning with it all.

We did, however, have the support of a lovely babysitter called Jenny. She would look after Flynn for me on Tuesday, and Daisy would go to school, so I'd make sure that any appointments to do with Seren were always booked on that day.

This particular Tuesday, I didn't have any appointments so Karl and I said we would spend the morning together, to reconnect, to cuddle, to just be.

We waved goodbye to Daisy and Flynn and were intending to drop Seren off at the workshop at 9.00 am. Seren, however, had different ideas and our beautiful morning to 'just be' was actually spent in utter turmoil.

After her hour-long crazy screaming fit, Seren had fallen asleep in the back of the car, so I leant over and put her seatbelt on and we drove home.

We stopped by the beach and as she slept, we got out of the car and sat looking at the ocean. We held each other and we cried, not a few tears, we cried a lot. I remember the breeze of the ocean and the sun beating down on us – two people, two best friends, two lovers who had been together for fifteen years who were now so lost, so confused and so sad.

The video

I showed the pediatrician the video and as we watched, I tried to be brave and not cry. But Seren's screaming was so haunting that tears rolled down my cheeks. It was a scream that no parent should ever have to hear when they are just loving, caring parents. The pediatrician said that we needed to have a plan.

He said we should continue with the medication; he felt that Seren had now 'learned behaviour' and it would take time to undo this.

He also stated that Risperidone wasn't a drug that he wanted Seren to be on for a long time, so he suggested she stay on it for six weeks and then we could look at behavioural classes and parenting classes.

He said we needed to have faith, break the cycle and continue with the medication. He also strongly suggested that we stop seeing the psychologist as he felt we were wasting our money and it was confusing for Seren.

So many decisions

We were in a complete haze, desperately and frantically trying different types of parenting. Although Seren's behaviour was much better at times, she was still having major meltdowns that were becoming more and more hard to handle.

It was during this time that we decided the best course of action would be to stop with the psychologist, as the pediatrician suggested. Seren was in the middle of another ten-week course with the psychologist, so we decided to let Seren keep going until the tenth session and then we would stop the sessions.

Karl advised the psychologist that we were now medicating Seren with Risperidone and using a time-out method. The psychologist felt that we would be better to use praise and teach Seren about emotional intelligence (having gone through it all, I can now say that I agree with her 100%). However, at the time, we were so lost and confused it was hard to work out which approach would be better. We had tried talking about emotions and that had seen Seren screaming and running off down the road. It hadn't worked, and although Seren was now medicated, we felt like we had a plan. The medication was helping and when it wasn't, we used the time-out method.

Karl had also told the psychologist that Seren was on Prozac, which was being used to treat her anxiety. The psychologist at the time had recommended Ritalin as she felt Seren was at the extreme end of ADHD. She also felt that Seren's anxiety could be treated with regular one-on-one cognitive behaviour therapy sessions.

Seren's teacher had praised the psychologist and had noted that Seren was starting to make friends and do better in school, but this had all changed when we went on the road trip. We used to feel that we would take one step forward and two steps back, and whenever her behaviour would be better, suddenly out if the blue it would take a turn for the worse.

Losing faith in the psychologist

The psychologist never seemed happy with the different approaches I tried with Seren. From diet to naturopathy, homoeopathy to marine plankton, time-out to emotional intelligence, she felt that I was going from one thing to another, confusing Seren and confusing the situation.

I asked if I could meet her for a chat – with all the stress, I felt like I needed to see a psychologist myself! We met for an hour and talked at length. We talked about my childhood, the fact that I was spanked as a child, and also the fact that I had smacked Seren on a couple of occasions. She felt that I had anger issues that needed to be sorted out, but she couldn't help me as she felt it would be a conflict of interest.

She recommended another psychologist who could give me a hand, as I may have ADHD too. However, I never made the call.

I think that I was starting to lose faith in this psychologist at this point.

How could seeing the two of us be a conflict of interest? Surely it could benefit both Seren and me?

We hadn't done as she had suggested and I am sure that she felt that if we just gave the Ritalin to Seren everything would be ok. I hadn't wanted to medicate her with Ritalin, but she was now on Prozac and Risperidone. I was starting to wonder what was worse and what was I doing?

I kept remembering what the pediatrician had told me: 'Prozac is one of the safest drugs to be used'. I also kept remembering that he had said to me, 'Seren will only be on Risperidone for six weeks and then we will start parenting and behaviour methods'. He knew of a counsellor who specialised in ADHD, helping parents and teachers. I was so excited about this. This was exactly what I had wanted!

Time for me to see a psychologist too?

I felt that the meeting with the psychologist had gone well; although, I did feel that she didn't really understand where I was going with it all. I probably seemed over-emotional, upset and stressed as I explained how I was trying my very best to cope with Seren's increasing outlandish behaviour.

I loved Seren with all I had, but during this time I didn't like her very much. It is very hard to like someone when they are taking you to the brink of despair. Karl felt the same, and to be honest we felt it from friends, from family and from the teachers.

Seren was difficult, she was hard to manage, she absolutely would not listen, she was mean, she was rude and she would lie. Don't get me wrong, my behaviour wasn't the best, and I don't think I was going to win the 'Mother of the Year Award' either.

I left the psychologist's office that day with some telephone numbers of other psychologists for me to see myself, but I was pretty sure that I wouldn't call them. I just didn't have the energy to speak to anyone else about this problem. I was starting to feel that maybe I should listen to the pediatrician and that maybe we were wasting our money!

Diary entries and correspondence during this time

5 February

Karl came home after taking Seren for her weekly appointment with the psychologist.

What he said crushed me and made me once again burst into tears like an emotional wreck.

'Seren is scared of Susy, and that it why she is having these anxiety attacks'. Karl said that Seren wasn't scared of me and that the problem was Seren. He said that at times I would shout at Seren like any parent, but I was a loving, caring mum.

I am literally at rock bottom.

I have tried everything and now this – it was my fault! I am angry, hurt and upset that we have gone down this route with the psychologist for nearly a year and now it is all my fault!

I asked Seren what had been said in today's sessions and she replied, 'Oh yeah, sorry Mummy, I kinda said that you had smacked me a couple of times and that I am scared of you, but I didn't mean to say it, the psychologist said it and I kinda agreed'.

So I asked, 'Are you afraid of me?'

'No, sorry Mummy, I just said it. I didn't mean it, sorry, love you!' And off she trotted, just like that. My world was shattered and Seren just skipped off.

So just like that we decided to take the pediatrician's advice and stop Seren seeing the psychologist.

5 February

Hi Diane,

I hope you had a wonderful holiday break. We've had a lovely time with family from the UK, but it's also been very trying with our little Seren. The pediatrician has diagnosed Seren with ADD and ODD (Oppositional Defiance Disorder). The ADD we can cope with and have resisted medicating, but the defiance was becoming very dangerous as Seren was starting to do things that could potentially harm her.

On this basis, three weeks ago the pediatrician prescribed Seren with a mood regulator and I have to say, it's been life-changing for us all, especially Seren. The only side effect is that she can become a little tired late afternoon. Seren will be on this medication for another five weeks and then we are going to start behavioural management classes instead of the medication. The pediatrician is hoping that the medication will break the behaviour cycle. Her behaviour was getting completely out of control, but we now feel we have a great pediatrician who understands Seren and we are making great progress.

It would be great to have a catch up in a couple of weeks to see how Seren is getting on.

Thanks so much Diane!

Love Susy xx

Hi Susy,

Great! Thanks for the information, and I would love to catch up next week when I have observed her a little more to get a feel for the change in her.

Diane xx

12 February

Hi Diane,

We reduced Seren's medication by half for the last three days and we really noticed a difference in her behaviour. The defiance started again and the hyperactivity seemed out of control yesterday. I am aware that the medication is making her drowsy so I'm not sure what to do about that. We are seeing the pediatrician in four weeks, but I'm going to email him to see if he has any suggestions.

When would you like to meet up next week so we can discuss Seren? Is Monday after school any good for you? I can have Daisy and Flynn looked after, so it will be easier.

Thanks so much, Diane!

Love Susy xx

Hi Susy,

I agree with you. Seren has been very unsettled these past few days and tired by 2.00 pm. Monday sounds great to meet with you. Can you see if there is a place in the diary through Debbie in the office?

You can email her to make it easy. Just say in your email it is to discuss Seren's emotional progress.

Diane xx

12 February

Seren isn't reading, in fact she is REFUSING to read. Seren is so hyper, she can't focus on her work. She is waking so early and can't sleep at night. She is up so late, I can't seem to get her to go to bed.

This is so hard.

13 February

Hi Ruth,

Thank you so much for your lovely email. A lot has happened since I last emailed. It's funny, I'm starting to feel that our emails are a little bit of therapy for me. It sometimes helps to write it all down to make sense of it all, so thank you so much for your kind words and interest – it means so much.

Seren has been on the medication for four weeks and although she is still very hyper, her defiance, moods and anger have been almost non-existent. She has still been getting a little drowsy in school for the last hour of the day, and even though the teachers have been so supportive, I was concerned about this.

We had almost convinced ourselves that as she was only taking a quarter of a tablet we could reduce it to an eighth and she would be fine.

Seren had an eighth of a tablet for three days, but her hyperactivity was out of control and she came home from school covered in bites on her arms (which she had done to herself). I calmly took her for a walk on the beach with Chip and we swam in the ocean. We talked about how she felt and she told me that her mind is 'cuckoo' and she has so many thoughts racing around her head, she doesn't know how to handle it. She told me that she is different to other people and she was born bad. I feel so sorry for her, as there must be something going on inside her head that we just can't see, so we don't really know how to help.

Her ADHD means that she is up now every morning at 5.00 am ... no wonder she's tired! Seren is also very hard to get to bed at night, although this is getting better. Anyway, we put her back on the normal medication yesterday and although she was still hyper she was a different child yesterday. She's now also doing excellently with her reading and is helping the younger children to read, which I'm so pleased with.

I'm meeting with Seren's teacher next week. I want to see how she is managing in school, as we still aren't medicating her for ADHD. I feel in time we will need to do this. Poor Seren, only seven years old and having to have medication. I feel awful about it. We are on the right track and we are making good progress with the medication so that can only be a good thing.

Karl is going snowboarding in Japan next week with his friends and brother, and one of my very good friends from the UK is coming to stay while he's away. I'm so excited and I think the break will do Karl and I the world of good!

We have found the Seren situation quite hard on our relationship and, as they say, absence makes the heart grow fonder!

I'm missing my friends a lot, especially Anna; I can't wait to see her in July!

Love Susy xx

16 February

Hi Susy,

The photos are great. It is so nice for me to picture where you are living and it looks like you have plenty of room for you all.

I have thought long and hard about your last email and I am happy that the medication she is taking is helping a little bit.

I do not know what else you can do because it seems like each situation is crisis management rather than long-term help.

At least Seren is now talking about things, but her self-esteem is really low so she needs masses of praise every day, and rewards for good behaviour often helps.

It must be so hard for you and Karl at the moment, but all you can do is try and come to terms with it all and not be too ambitious with your plans for family outings and events. Keep to a good routine.

Keep in touch and I will always be thinking about you.

Love Ruth

My relationship with Ruth

During this whole journey, I bared so much of my soul to Ruth. She was a wonderful, wise lady who had three children of her own and had five grand-children who were all excelling in life. They were Grade A students going to Oxford and Cambridge universities. Ruth's children had gone to boarding school and later on had all gone to university. Her children lived in Paris, London and Germany, and I guess I aspired that one day my children could be successful just like Ruth's children.

I loved to chat with Ruth. I somehow felt that she would have the answers. I really valued Ruth's advice and I looked forward to her emails of support each month. Some of Ruth's advice I should have listened to a lot more, for instance, 'family outings and events'. I really wished that I had remembered these words of wisdom before booking a last minute holiday to Phuket in Thailand. I wish that I had read back through my diary before we booked this holiday, I should have realised that Seren wouldn't cope.

When I was younger, my family had a holiday home in Wales, at a caravan park at the edge of the most beautiful beach in a place called Nefyn. We would go down to the caravan whenever we could. I had friends there and I loved the familiar smells of the caravan, the views of the beach, the different birds, and the absolute quietness of the little Welsh village in the middle of nowhere. We had the holiday home until Seren was a baby, so it was beautiful being able to take Seren down to our little holiday home haven too.

I might have acted like Seren if my parents had taken me all over the place. Who knows? For some kids they are fine, but for many with ADHD and anxiety, the thought of travelling to a new place fills them with dread and their behaviour starts to nosedive again. Seren's did as soon as we set foot in Phuket!

More worrying behaviours

Days before we left for Thailand, I went to see the pediatrician about Seren because I was worried about some of her behaviours. The pediatrician had said that she would only be on Risperidone for six weeks, but it had now been eight weeks and this concerned me, as I knew that it was a strong medication.

Many children are on this medication for years, and I am sure they are fine. However, many are not fine as they suffer from side effects, sometimes even after the drug has been discontinued. I was starting to notice side effects in Seren that I was not happy with at all, and I started to notice them after about six weeks.

Seren had put on weight after we started her on the medication. As a heath conscious mum, this did worry me but I tried to pretend that it didn't. Seren literally couldn't stop eating; she would eat her food, then finish Daisy's, then Flynn's and would still be hungry. I couldn't seem to fill her up and this worried me I as wondered what the medication was doing to her.

I tried not to worry too much, though, as her behaviour had been better. What really did concern me though was the fact that Seren was starting to grow hairs on her legs, hairs that she should only have when a little girl starts puberty. She was also starting to get spots on her chin and her little non-existent breasts, which you would expect for a seven-year-old, were starting to swell!

I assessed it for a week or so and then decided to go and chat with the pediatrician again. (I am sure he must have been sick of me!) I talked about all the physical changes that were happening to Seren but also some emotional changes that were happening to her, which had also been noted by Seren's teacher.

Seren had started to show an interest in boys. She would chase them all day and would write in her notebook about how much she loved them. This behaviour was so weird because it only began when Seren started taking Risperidone. She also started to dance very provocatively, often talking like a baby. And she was still talking about death regularly.

I knew in my heart of hearts that it was down to the medication and that it was doing something to my little girl. Even though there were positive changes in her behaviour, these side effects could have grave consequences if we continued with the medication.

The pediatrician was very honest and said that he thought Seren was going through 'promiscuous puberty'. Promiscuous puberty is one of the many side effects of Risperidone. Right away, I knew that I was going to have to go back to the never-ending nightmare of bad behaviour because there was no way that I would allow my seven year old to start going through puberty.

The pediatrician suggested taking Seren off the medication. He also felt that because she was on such a low dose, it should be easy just to stop it immediately.

Can you imagine what would be happening to Seren if she had had the recommended dose? I was only giving her a quarter of the recommended dose, yet in six short weeks my seven-year-old daughter was starting to go through puberty! I was actually petrified that I had done some damage to Seren's little body; her little body that I had grown in my womb eagerly for nine months.

I had done everything right in my pregnancy. When she was born, I had breastfed her, then weaned her on only home-made organic food. And I had only ever used natural organic products on her. We had lived in the country in the UK, grown our vegetables, had chickens, and yet here I was giving my daughter mind-altering, hormone-altering drugs?

What has happened? What sort of mum am I now? What am I doing to her?

I hated myself. I hated who I had become and I felt like such a failure.

I followed other mums on Instagram and they seemed to have it together – happy children, happy homes, happy lives. I guess my life must have resembled that if they looked at my account, but in reality, it was a very different story. I feared the worst for Seren and I feared the worst for our little family.

I suggested to the pediatrician that we pretend to carry on giving Seren the medication, as a placebo. Overall her behaviour had been so much better and calmer since taking the drug. We had seen some meltdowns but there had been a significant change from where we had started.

I could always tell when Seren's behaviour was better as there wouldn't be any diary entries in my book about her. During the eight weeks that Seren was taking Risperidone, I only updated my journal four times! During the bad times, I would write in the diary every day. Writing all the things that had happened during the day was my source of comfort and escape. I guess it was some therapy, and believe me I needed lots of it!

Yes, another 'hell-i-day'

As planned, we went to Thailand. However, the day after we arrived, I noticed that Daisy and Flynn had spots all over their hands and feet! I took them to the doctors and they confirmed what I thought – 'hand, foot and mouth disease'. Well that was the Kids Club out of the window for those two! Seren would go to Kids Club most mornings, and she said she had lots of fun; however, it wasn't too long before they called us in to say they were struggling with her.

I still wasn't really telling anyone that Seren had ADHD, but I did tell the Kids Club and they thanked me for letting them know as they could manage her differently. I wondered what it was that they were going to do to 'manage her differently', and I hoped that they could tell me as I didn't have a clue how to parent her!

Diary entry during this time

12 April
It started on day two of the holiday. Running away, hiding, defiant, abusive, rude. Losing her all the time. She is never listening to me. Ignoring me when I call her, horrendous!!!!!!!! I tell her off and put her on time-out, and then she pulls her knickers down and trumps in Karl's face. She deliberately tries to upset me if I'm worried about

something. We watched her interact with people in the pool. Even a boy had enough of her antics and kicked her into the pool. She's been an absolute nightmare. Help!!! :-(

At the end of my tether

To say I was at the end of my tether was an understatement. Life had become so hard. I desperately wanted to have a normal life and live a normal family life, but I was also having inner turmoil with myself because I didn't want Seren medicated.

I knew things had to change. We had tried different types of medication with Seren and still her behaviour was out of control. I have to say that on this holiday, her behaviour was unbearable, and her defiance was out of control. However, more than that, her hyperactivity was ridiculous and so was her impulsivity.

We made a conscious decision during this holiday that we would do with Seren what my dad had done with me (no, not a mighty one), but the same type of holiday each year. We would go camping, caravanning, and ensure familiarity, and do this in Australia. We were so lucky to live in one of the most amazing countries and we intended to enjoy it!

We hadn't been on many holidays for the last couple of years in the UK. We had Daisy and Flynn quite close together, and Karl was working such long hours that holidays took a bit of a back burner. When we came to Australia, Karl had some time at home and we decided that, whenever we could, we would use this time to go on a couple of holidays.

Karl, Daisy and Flynn had an excellent time, and I think Seren did, but it became a research holiday for me. We would put the kids to bed at around 8.00 pm, Karl would watch a movie and then I would research ADHD.

I was determined to find another way, there had to be! Maybe the diet wasn't right, maybe she was deficient in something, maybe she had too much lead or copper in her system, perhaps it was the parenting? Here I went again ... but I was convinced that I was missing something!

Shouting and the occasional smack definitely wasn't helping, and it was making me become further and further from the Instagram mums who seemed to have the perfect children only playing with wooden toys, homeschooling, and weaving creations with branches they had found in the woods or on the beach.

I wanted to be that mum so much. I knew I could be that mum! Ok, maybe the weaving was a step too far, and definitely the homeschooling (I don't think I have the patience), but the wooden toys – check.

I dreamt that one day the perfect Instagram mums would suddenly show a picture of chaos or a messy house or kids screaming or proclaim suddenly, 'My life with ADHD'. But none one of them did and so I found myself overcome with self-hatred, hating what I had become and who I was.

Life isn't that perfect and although it may have seemed like that to my friends and family in the UK, with all the beautiful pictures of the ocean and hashtagging about love and family and happiness, I was actually in the middle of a breakdown and didn't know where to turn!

Chapter Seven

Making peace with medication
(for now anyway)

I don't think I ever really made peace with medication. I tried to. I desperately tried to. I really wanted a miracle. I wanted to find a 'dream' medication – one that wouldn't harm Seren long-term or give her side effects. But I came to realise that this type of medication – just like the pot of gold at the end of the rainbow – didn't exist.

We arrived home from Thailand, and I organised an appointment with the pediatrician. (Now there's a change!) We also arranged for Seren's friend Tilly to come over and stay for the weekend. Seren had lots of friends in the UK, but she hadn't made any friends in Australia, even though we had lived here now for fourteen months. She talked about her best friends in her new school but whenever I saw them together, they seemed quite annoyed with her.

Seren had only been invited to one party since we moved here and she hadn't been invited to any play dates. I felt so sad for her as Seren had lots of friends in the UK.

I always wondered what life would have been like if we had stayed in the UK. *Would friends have stopped asking her for play dates? Would she not have been invited to parties anymore? Would she have had the same problems in the UK as she was having here? Was this just happening to Seren because she had ADHD? Or was it because we had moved to a new country and a new type of schooling?*

I asked myself these questions over and over again, overthinking the whole thing. I drove myself mad.

Seren's friend Tilly

When I was eighteen, I had a friend called Mike. He had spent most of his twenties and thirties living abroad, so I hadn't seen him for years. He moved to Perth a couple of years before we did, and he lived there with his adorable family. I used to love looking at all his photos – his life looked idyllic.

Two years before we moved, we came to Perth for a family holiday and Mike invited us over for lunch. We met his wife, Angie, who was due any day with their third baby, and his two gorgeous daughters, Tilly and Poppy. They told us all about their adventures 'Down Under', as we relaxed, ate lunch and watched the kids play in the pool.

Seren was four at the time, and Tilly was five, but even then we noticed how similar they were. The two of them seemed to strike up a friendship straightaway, and Seren would often talk about 'Tilly in Australia'.

When we moved to Australia, Angie became such an incredible support, giving me help, advice and tips on suburbs, schools and the 'Ozzie' way of life. During one particular get-together at our house, I was giving Seren iron and fish oils as they arrived. Angie told me that she also gave those to Tilly and then went on to explain how Tilly had been diagnosed with ADHD a year ago.

We hardly told a soul about Seren's own diagnosis, especially here in Perth, so to have friends who were going through a similar thing felt like such a relief. I hugged Angie so tight and tears welled in my eyes as I told how Seren had just been diagnosed with ADHD too.

Mike and Angie have become such good friends and their advice and support has been invaluable over the last eighteen months. Tilly, like Seren, also struggles with anxiety and they have lots of similarities. Some days when we get together, Seren's behaviour is worse and sometimes it's Tilly's. However, we never judge each other. We only give love and support to one another, at times even laughing together at the craziness of it all.

A couple of days after we arrived back from Thailand, Karl collected Tilly and then took Seren and Tilly out for pizza, while I stayed at home with Daisy and Flynn. Karl said Seren was wild. She wasn't able to sit at the table and eat her dinner, and she kept getting up from her seat and running around the restaurant while Tilly sat calmly and ate her pizza. He couldn't believe how out of control and crazy Seren was; yet Tilly's behaviour was amazing.

When the girls got home, they ran upstairs to play in Seren's room, taking Chip, the dog, with them. Suddenly we heard Chip yelp, followed by Tilly screaming, 'Karl, quick help!'

Karl ran up the stairs and started yelling at Seren. I quickly followed upstairs and saw Karl cradling Chip. Next to him, Seren was laughing like a wild child without a care in the world. Seren had put Chip on the top bunk bed and then couldn't work out how to get Chip down, so she decided to throw him off the top bunk. Tilly looked pale and was positively shocked and upset, but Seren seemed so crazy that she couldn't even see what she had done wrong. She didn't seem at all bothered and had no empathy whatsoever.

It was also during this weekend that Seren cut some of her hair off. She had her hair braided in Thailand, and so I had explained to her that she would have to take them out before school on Monday. Seren was about to have a shower and I was bathing Flynn and Daisy. She saw that I was busy and couldn't help with her braids, so she said, 'Mummy, don't worry, I can do it'.

I thought it was really sweet, so I agreed and she took herself upstairs into her bedroom. When Seren came back downstairs, she'd removed about half of the braids. I took the rest out while keeping an eye on Daisy and Flynn in the bath. I hadn't even noticed the disaster that had happened upstairs and it was only when Tilly said, 'Seren, why is your hair like that?' that I noticed what she had done. I gasped as I realised that Seren had not undone the braids that night, she had cut them off, at the roots! The crown of her beautiful blonde long hair now resembled a tennis ball; tears once again fell from my face.

We knew that we had to do something, and that something quickly. Seren was doing such impulsive things that we now feared the worst. What made me so upset and angry was that she had been on medication for eight weeks and it was supposed to break the cycle. Not only had it failed to break the cycle, but Seren's behaviour was now a million times worse.

Tilly was on ADHD medication, and after seeing how calm and how well behaved she was, we felt that maybe medicating Seren for her ADHD would be the way forward.

Diary entries during this time

25 April

Seren's behaviour is so crazy and wild that the school can't teach her anymore. She is losing friends and even threw Chip off the top bunk today.

We are again at breaking point – the defiance isn't that bad anymore, but she is so crazy that she is unaware what she is doing.

The ADHD has reached record levels and, despite all our efforts, we now have no choice but to medicate. We need to medicate her for the next few days, as she has once more become a danger to herself and the family. It's very sad, but I feel we have no choice. We have tried everything and I am now at the end of my tether. It's time to medicate and I'm completely comfortable with the decision. :-)

26 April

We woke up and Seren was crazy! Decided to give her some Risperidone, but it made her sleepy. She slept all morning. It calmed her down so much, so she was manageable.

I have decided to go and get myself diagnosed with ADHD. I can then start a strategy for myself, as I need to be in a good place so I can be a good mum for Seren.

I am going to suggest Strattera to the pediatrician. It seems to be working for Tilly and I like the fact that it isn't a stimulant. Anyway, I will see what he says.

Plan
- Medicate
- Seren to see a regular counsellor – CBT to help her understand and cope
- School holidays – Camp Australia for consistency
- Maybe Tilly and Seren could go together?
- Regular play dates with Tilly
- Susy – get a diagnosis and manage through medication
- maybe on bad days, meditation, yoga etc. and regular counselling or me
- Seren – music, swimming, sports, arts etc.

Utter chaos!

When I read these diary entries, I see that I was in complete and utter chaos management and I had no idea how to cope with Seren's behaviour. It did seem like I was chopping and changing everything, but I was a desperate mother going through an absolute battle with myself on a daily basis. Medicate or not medicate? Time-out or praise the good?

Every expert I spoke to, every book I read, every blog, podcast or video all had conflicting advice. I wished that there was some sort of plan, some sort of step-by-step guide to try before jumping around and trying all these different medications. Plus, there were the added statements such as – 'ADHD isn't real', 'ADHD is made up', 'ADHD is a mental illness', 'ADHD is a superpower'. It was during this time that I realised that ADHD is possibly one of the biggest controversies of our time – the world is split on how it should be managed by parents, schools and society. No wonder I chopped and changed my mind so much!

I had the school saying to me on a daily basis that they were unable to teach her. The choir teacher even had to kindly ask Seren to leave because she was so disruptive.

I was starting to think that it was my fault and maybe I had ADHD and needed medication. I looked into my family tree and saw that on both sides there were problems with depression and addiction.

Maybe it is me? Was it's my fault? My genes?

But I wasn't a bad mum. I had two other normal, great, well-behaved children.

Why am I blaming myself? Who am I?

I didn't know anymore. I was lost in the chaos.

We had tried everything!

We tried every natural alternative going other than neurofeedback, which I did look into, and although it was expensive, I was prepared to try anything. I had contacted a neurofeedback clinic in Perth and had a long chat with them. They reassured me how successful it was and I asked for references before we made the decision.

They advised me they would send me some contact numbers of parents who had success for their ADHD children. They never got back to me, so I figured that was my answer. The pediatrician also felt that neurofeedback would be a waste of money and at this point we had spent thousands of dollars!

We had tried medication, which had been successful, but Seren had experienced terrible side effects and, if we continued, we could change her forever. Also, the plan to break the cycle had not worked. The pediatrician felt that Seren would only need to be on this medication for six weeks and that's all we would need. As I have mentioned previously, sadly, when she came off the medication after eight weeks, her behaviour was worse than ever.

I still wonder to this day – how could I have given Seren Risperidone again after I knew of the side effects? I ask myself this question so many times, and the answer is simple

... Desperation.

I was not well

It was during this time that I started to realise that all was not well in the 'Susy camp'. My mind raced continually, all I thought about was ADHD. I lived, breathed and dreamed about ADHD, about Seren, about the school, and my thoughts became more and more dramatic. I couldn't think about anything else, all I talked about was Seren or ADHD or medication. I was confused and scared and out of my depth.

One night, when I was talking to Billy and Lucy, they could see how stressed I was and what it was doing to our family. Billy told me about a friend that he worked for whose son had been diagnosed with ADHD, and how they had decided to medicate him with Ritalin. For them it had been a lifesaver and their son was now studying at university. I started to hear more positive stories about how medication had saved children and saved families, and I was starting to become more open-minded to it.

Maybe the psychologist was right. Maybe the problem was me? Maybe I was just making the whole situation worse because I didn't want to give Seren a stimulant medication, but maybe she really needed it. Maybe I had just prolonged the pain and made everything worse?

Seren was unable to concentrate at home or at school. She was impulsive, hyper, defiant, angry and emotional, and I now needed to grow some big shoulders, grow a pair, and man up!

Diary entries and correspondence during this time

28 April

Seren and I saw the pediatrician yesterday and we both decided that Ritalin would be the way forward. We are going to gradually increase the daily dose, so as of tomorrow she will be on 2 x daily doses, one at breakfast and one at lunchtime.

Already we see a much better improvement. Please let this work! I've decided not to give her the 25 mg, but give her 20 mg; we can always increase it if we need to.

I'm putting all my fears aside and realising that this will be the best way forward for Seren. I am trying to let her play after school for thirty mins per day so she gets some daily exercise. I feel this will help her. Her appetite seems ok actually, so I am pleased about this. She is sleeping fine and all is well in the world. I am keeping up with the supplements too!

2 May

Hi Ruth,

How are you all? We are good and gearing up to coming back to the UK in July.

I think you said you are away on 17th? We will come and see you before then. It's very exciting!

Flynn is starting to say more words now and plays really well with Daisy – endless games of mummy and daddy. I love watching them play! They both love Daddy and fight over him; it's amusing to watch! Seren's behaviour hasn't been great and unfortunately she hasn't been doing great at school either. Two incidents last weekend prompted us to medicate her for ADHD. We are all in a good place with it and I've finally made peace with the decision.

Seren only started taking it last week so we are hoping that it's going to really help her. We are also starting CBT sessions next week and I'm hoping that this will help her, and us all, greatly too. We're not sure if Montessori education is the best for Seren going forward, so we are starting to look at other options now too. I've read heaps of books and have invested so much time into researching ADHD; I probably could write a book on it now!

We still love living here. We spend a lot of time down at the beach and outside, and I feel this is a godsend for Seren as she has boundless energy! She is starting to love books, which I'm so pleased about. She listens to her audio books before school and before bed when doing her craft and drawing, which she loves. She's very creative, very kind and has such confidence when she's on the stage singing and dancing. Karl is great ... he's still working out which direction his life is going, but things are starting to happen, so this is exciting!

I'm starting to think about what I would like to do in the future too. It's all good!

I'm starting to make some lovely friends here, which is helping with the homesickness.

Hope all is great with you guys! When did you say the tenants were away? We would love to pop in and say hello!

Lots of love to you both.

Love Susy xx

Hi Susy,

It looks like you enjoyed your Thailand holiday from the Facebook photos.

I am sorry to hear that Seren needs the ADHD medication, but I'm glad in a way, as I know it will settle her down. From my experience, perhaps when she is older, late teens, she can choose when to take it or have a spell off it. A great friend of Louise's son was diagnosed when he was fourteen and now he is really good and just uses the medication when he is taking exams and really needs to concentrate. He is at Exeter uni reading psychology, and all his best work is done when he does not take the medication.

Reading for Seren could become her escape, which is so important. Maybe a more structured school discipline will suit her. Personally, I have never been a fan of the Montessori system.

It will be great to see you in July. The tenants are away from either the 4th or 5th July. Friends are so important all through your life, but it does take time to find the ones with the same values of life as yours. Flynn and Daisy are going to be such good pals and they look so sweet in the photos.

Thinking about you lots.

Love Ruth xx

3 May

Seren has told me that she hasn't been getting any of her privileges in school. She has to do work all day, isn't allowed to play outside and isn't allowed to spend time with her friends. She doesn't understand what she has done wrong. I'm starting to feel like the Montessori education isn't working for Seren. :-(

Seren seems really anxious, very teary and she can't cope with noise.

I feel so sorry for her and I feel so sorry for us as a family. I'm really struggling to cope. I am feeling very depressed and cut off from everyone. I feel so sad ... :-(

5 May

Seren's behaviour is wild! She wakes up and literally screams. She doesn't do any of her tasks and runs around the house whipping everyone into a frenzy.

She has her breakfast and takes her Ritalin and then after forty minutes she can function, do her jobs and she leaves the house calmly.

Daddy collected her from school after choir. He told her that he was going to take her skateboarding and for dinner. Seren was defiant and her behaviour was awful while they were out together. She was running away, hiding, defiant, screaming and not doing as she was told. Her behaviour sometimes is very unnerving. I sometimes worry that it's not ADHD but something much worse.

Sometimes when Seren sleeps in my bed, she acts oddly. I sometimes feel that in the future I'm not sure what she is capable of. I hope I'm wrong and I'm just being silly. My dad has seen it too and it also made him feel very uncomfortable. I hope I'm wrong. I really do hope it's just ADHD!

6 May

Seren woke up this morning really late. We found this helped the rest of us because it was harmonious and happy. Seren went to school feeling great! But she didn't drink water or eat all day and seemed wired when I picked her up from school. She played after school in the park with her friends but seemed distant and depressed. She wouldn't let me engage in any conversations with people. We all got in the car and then she started kicking the back of Flynn's seat. She said she'd had a horrible day in school. She started screaming, saying she hates her name and had hidden underneath a chair in school. She went on to say that she had worked really hard in school.

Seren often talks like a baby and goes from one extreme to another. She is defiant and hyper and then she starts being overly loving, but it just feels uncomfortable.

I sometimes wonder if it really is ADHD. Seren pretended to cut her throat with her knife and fork at dinner, and Daisy got upset and talked about this when she went to bed later on with Daddy.

7 May

Seren poured porridge all over the breakfast bar and refused to get dressed and follow any instructions today.

On Risperidone, Seren would do all her morning tasks, but now she doesn't do anything. She is defiant, anxious; she lies and is unable to carry out simple instructions, even when on Ritalin. Her anxiety seems worse than ever. This morning she was lying on the breakfast bar as we were trying to eat breakfast. I asked her three times to get down but she refused. I sent her on time-out; she didn't go. I then shouted at her and she ran off hysterically screaming. :-(

The only thing that has ever worked is Risperidone, but I don't want her going back on that; however, I am not sure the Ritalin is right for her either?

Initial side effects of Ritalin

Not only was her behaviour not really improving while on the Ritalin, there were some other side effects we noticed. After school, Seren would only want to watch TV. She didn't seem to have the energy to do anything else, which was so unlike her. She would also just sit there and bite the insides of the mouth, gurn, and she developed a tic, which meant she would move her head up and down constantly, and sometimes her arms and legs would intermittently start moving too. This became worse over time. Her lunch box was untouched and her water bottle was still full to the brim.

How can a medication work effectively when my seven-year-old isn't eating or drinking all day?

We now have so much information and data available to us; we know how important food is to our brains as well as to our bodies. We are aware how deficient our diets are of essential nutrients and vitamins, and we are told how important gut health is, and how it's linked to mental health.

How then could it be right for Seren long-term or even short-term to not be eating or drinking all day?

Behavioural lessons

It was time to start with some behavioural lessons! I had seen a leaflet in the pediatrician's office months ago and I had asked him about it many times. He had talked about having behavioural sessions with Seren after we managed her behaviour when she was taking Risperidone.

I personally still feel that it is wrong to prescribe medication before a family assessment of some sort occurs. *What if there are major problems in the family? What if there is abuse? Mental illness? Alcohol or drug addiction? Or even just a lack or parenting, wouldn't it be better to look at this first before medication? I know that they do this in countries in Europe, so why not here?*

The pediatrician had said that we had to sort out Seren's behaviour first, then we had to find the right medication, and then start on the behavioural classes. We had tried three different types of medication and Seren's behaviour was getting worse; we couldn't go back to Risperidone, even though he had suggested it.

I honestly couldn't be responsible for destroying a little girl's life, a child's future – I just couldn't do it, no matter how hard things became.

Chapter Eight

Sensory tents and jam jars

Squidgy toys, fairy lights, doggy toys, light up teddies, pillows, soft cushions and blankets with tassels – well they do say that 'God loves a trier'! Maybe if we tried everything, the Universe would send us a miracle?

The counsellor specialised in ADHD in both children and adults. She had first-hand experience with ADHD with her own children, and she ran workshops and private sessions. I wasn't sure why the pediatrician hadn't set this up. He had mentioned it many times and yet, despite my efforts, he still hadn't organised anything.

Working together

I had one of the behavioural lessons leaflets sitting on the fridge and I looked at it daily. The more I looked at it, the more I felt it was time to try these lessons.

We had systemically tried everything but this we hadn't. Not only would it just involve the family and the counsellor, the counsellor would also work with the school. I felt that if we could all work together, we would have a much better outcome for Seren, and it would be consistent.

Karen had talked about how they did things in the UK. She said that the pediatricians, psychologists, parents and the school would all work together to help the child. She said we needed a 'team Seren'. There didn't seem to be that kind of support here in Perth, everyone seemed to work individually, and I feel that this is one of the reasons why I was struggling.

No-one seemed to work together, cross-referencing and communicating, it all seemed to be very 'cloak and danger'. And that is probably why I was completely out of my depth with it all.

The importance of a team

I remember watching a program from the UK, which was called *Born Naughty*. Karen had told me about it, and Olivia had emailed me to say that she thought I should watch it.

What I loved about the TV show was that they had a team of experts who monitored the child through their home life, in school and also in a play setting with other children. The team involved a psychiatrist, psychologist and a pediatrician. Over the course of a few weeks, they all assessed the child and then came to a conclusion together – diagnosing the child.

I thought this was a wonderful idea and would have benefitted Seren. I, on the other hand, was haphazardly going from one expert to another, reading books and spending hours on the internet, trying to work out what was wrong with Seren. Thoughts whirled around my mind constantly.

Did Seren have ADHD?

What if Seren was on the autistic spectrum?

What if she had schizophrenia; she tells me her brain told her to be naughty?

Was it conduct disorder?

Was it something to do with vaccinations when she was younger?

Did she have too many metals in her body?

Too much lead, too much copper?

My mind wondered and my thoughts drove me crazy! My dad once told me, 'Susy, it's not the snake that kills you, it's chasing that sucker that drives the poison to the heart'. This quote makes total sense, but it's so hard to put into practice.

I knew that I was driving the poison to my heart and destroying myself with my negative, constant thoughts, but no matter how hard I tried, I couldn't switch them off!

Meeting the counsellor

Seren was on stimulant medication when I met with the counsellor. She would constantly smack her lips, chew her mouth, gurn, and her pupils were so dilated that we couldn't see her beautiful blue eyes. However, on the flip side, she was less fidgety, was able to sit down, look the counsellor in the eyes and talk to her calmly about how she felt. This was something that would have been impossible before now.

The counsellor encouraged me to focus on the positives. If Seren was very good at something, I was to allow her to channel her energies into this, as it would increase her self-esteem. Often ADHD kids have a very low opinion of themselves.

Notes from the meeting with the counsellor 7 May

- Focus on positives
- Praise and rewards
- Pay pocket money at the beginning of the week
- Pocket money in a jar
- 'Magic 1,2,3'
- Smiling minds app
- Audio in the car – iPod
- Sensory tent – time-in instead of time-out
- Heavy wheat pack to be used when sitting down
- Tent – reject shop, fill it with squishy balls, doggy chew toys, velvet cushions, sensory things.

The counsellor explained that she felt 'Magic 1,2,3' would be better for Seren as opposed to 'instant time-out' for not doing as she was told. She explained that the brain of someone with ADHD is very different as they are unable to 'toggle' when they are put in time-out. Therefore, the time-out doesn't do anything other than cause more anxiety in the child, which then makes the ADHD worse. 'Toggle' in layman terms means the process of thoughts between different parts of the brain. For example, many children when put on time-out will eventually stop that behaviour, as their brain will associate the time-out with the bad behaviour.

The counsellor explained that as the frontal part of the brain in ADHD children works differently, often these messages are not received properly and the child doesn't understand why they have been put in time-out. All it actually does is increase anxiety and cause the child to become more defiant to protect themselves. It made complete sense, and I wondered why I had never read that before in any book or website.

The counsellor then said the ultimate words that made me feel so safe and happy, and I really felt that we were finally in safe hands! She said that what we needed to do was to make a 'team Seren'! She said she would write a report to the pediatrician and let him know everything she had suggested.

I also vented to her my anxiety that I didn't feel the Ritalin was working for Seren, and we discussed that the only medication that had worked for Seren was the Risperidone. The counsellor then suggested Dextroamphetamine, telling me that it could often work better than the Ritalin.

She also explained to Seren all about ADHD, drawing a diagram and explaining to her that the front part of her brain worked differently to other people's brains. She explained through a drawing that there were two parts to the frontal part of the brain and that with ADHD kids they weren't very good at getting the message across, but medication helps them to talk.

Seren listened intently and asked several questions. We had been going through the process with Seren for the last year, but we had never discussed what was different with Seren. She just felt that she was 'born naughty'.

Finally, with the counsellor's explanations, it felt like we were allowing Seren to own who she was. This still sat uncomfortably with me, though. I hated watching my daughter sit twitching and gurning with the counsellor as they explained to her that she was different to other children.

The counsellor was beautiful and caring and, out of all of the experts that we had seen, she was the best. She had a warm, caring manner, and she gave me some advice that changed the course of our path, and for that, I am truly grateful.

Time-in items

When we left the meeting that day, I dropped Seren back off at school and I immediately went to the shops to buy all the 'time-in' items that the counsellor had recommended. I bought squishy toys, fairy lights, a jam jar, and then went to the post office and exchanged ten dollars for 100 ten cent coins that I then put in the jam jar for a 'reward system' for both Seren and Daisy.

I grabbed a little tent and set it up in the guest room with lots of cushions and things for Seren to play with. It would help to keep her entertained and help her calm down – it was like a sensory tent.

I filled the jar with all the coins and then that afternoon showed Seren the tent and the jar, and we had a little chat about how things were going to be from now on.

'Mummy's making some changes. No more time-outs, we are instead going to have "time-ins" and we are going back to "Magic 1,2,3".'

Did Seren ever use her sensory tent? No. But Daisy and Flynn had a superb time in it and it became Chip's new dog basket, so at least it was used!

The money in the jar idea was great. I didn't do it exactly as the counsellor had suggested, I have tweaked it a few times since then, and it works slightly differently for Daisy and Seren as they are very different children. It is still one of the best forms of reward that I have found and the best thing is that it's so easy to use. I can use it when we are out and it even goes on holiday with us, so I would say those little glass jam jars are now a big part of the family! This is the system that I mentioned in Chapter 4.

Diary entry during this time

8 May

I met with Seren's teacher today and she felt the same as me – Seren's defiance is worse than ever! She is agitated, paranoid, scared and hyper- sensitive! They were unable to teach her and she was unable to play with her friends.

When I collected her that night, Seren couldn't even bear anyone talking! She was out of control, running off, hiding etc.

Anxiety now a big problem

The meeting with Seren's teacher confirmed how I was feeling. The teacher also felt that while Seren's focus and concentration were better, she was becoming anxious and 'zoned out'. She talked about how Seren would be charming in the morning and would do a lot of schoolwork because she was more focused and calm. Lunchtimes were fine, Seren would play with her friends, but after she took her lunch dose of Ritalin, her pupils would dilate so much that the teacher could hardly see the blue in her eyes.

Seren would become very agitated and she was very sensitive to noise, sometimes hiding under tables or hiding in the toilets. It was during these few days that Seren tried to escape from school. She had run out of class and had climbed onto the fence, refusing to come down even when told to by her teacher. Seren never told me about any of these instances, and I only ever found out from her teacher as we conversed continually through email about Seren's behaviour.

Seren was taking Ritalin SA, which was the shorter-acting medication that would last for about four hours. She took one dose in the morning, and then she would take her 'lunchtime' dose that would last another four hours. This was conveniently packed into Seren's lunch box and it sat in a little tablet box cushioned around her 'healthy eating' carrot sticks, hummus, and apple and orange slices.

Biscuits and chocolates weren't allowed in her lunch box, but a medicated speed tablet – that was completely fine!

After the meeting with Seren's teacher on Friday, Karl and I decided that the Ritalin definitely wasn't working. I remember driving home from school that afternoon with all the kids in the car; it was the usual get up – Flynn was crying and shouting, and Daisy was incessantly talking. This was quite normal and we were all used to it, but this particular day Seren started screaming and holding her ears, saying, 'Make it stop. Make it stop'. She started hitting her head and then kicking the back of Flynn's chair. She was so upset and began rocking to comfort herself.

How could this medication possibly be working?

There have been so many studies done to prove that medication isn't enough and that once the children stop taking the medication, often the behaviour starts again. Then the parents have no option other than to go back to the medication.

Did it make Seren's behaviour better? Yes, she was able to sit and do her work and her teachers felt she was able to concentrate better.

Did it help Seren to focus better? Yes, she once came home from school and read a whole book, before that we could barely get her to read one page without her collapsing into an uncontrollable screaming fit.

But how did she feel? How was it making her feel? She seemed very anxious, frightened, and her emotions were all over the place. She seemed dead behind the eyes and seeing her pupils dilated, watching her unable to eat, and watching her gurning while she chewed her mouth was just too upsetting for me to watch. As I have mentioned briefly before, Seren also developed a tic and this took months to subside after she finished taking Ritalin. The pediatrician assured me that it wasn't because of the medication; however, I knew it was as it started when she began taking Ritalin. It finally stopped when she had an iron transfusion, but I will come to this in more detail later.

I am not judging anyone who medicates their children; I am simply expressing how it made me feel as Seren's mum.

Medicated speed allowed at school

I know some people would say that Ritalin and other such stimulant drugs aren't the same as speed, and I would 100% agree. I remember taking speed in my youth. I have heard that Ritalin is actually much better and cleaner as it hasn't been cut with anything such as bleach, horse tranquilliser or rat poison!

In fact, I think that this is the reason why so many youngsters are getting high on prescription medications – they are pretty good and often a lot better than the drugs you buy off the streets. And the best bit – they don't need to buy them from dealers off the streets. They can buy these drugs from their friends who have a cupboard full of them and have been using them since they were younger for their ADHD.

Nuts aren't allowed in schools, but soft drinks, cakes, biscuits, chocolate and sweets are allowed, even though we have an obesity crisis in Australia. If you are caught smoking marijuana in school, you will be suspended or expelled, but taking medicated speed, well that's absolutely fine!

One of my friends has a daughter who has a nut allergy, so I know how important it is not to have nuts in school. I get it, but I have learnt that sugar, preservatives and additives can also affect some children's behaviour so why are these still available in schools and why isn't the government doing more about this issue?

As simple as supplements

I once watched a TED talk presented by Julia Rucklidge, a leading psychologist in New Zealand. She had done studies on children and adults who were on medication for mental illnesses such as depression, ADHD and bipolar.

She discovered that the children and adults were deficient in various vitamins and nutrients and when she gave them very specific supplements, their symptoms were less and they didn't need to take medication anymore.

She took a group of children with various diagnoses, half of them were medicated and half of them weren't. What she discovered was that once they grew into adulthood, the ones who were medicated as children often ended up having more problems than the children who weren't medicated. Their mental illness even became worse, often changing from ADHD to bipolar or schizophrenia.

She strongly felt that if medication for mental illness was working, then why was depression and mental illness rising not decreasing? She felt that the government needed to change their approach and look at different types of approaches to treating mental illness.[18]

I only watched this after we had stopped medicating Seren, but at the time of medicating her, my only comfort and sanity was the medical profession. I had no-one else to turn to, or trust or believe, so I did what was suggested and medicated Seren.

Could it be worse than ADHD?

As I have mentioned previously, I had also become frightened that Seren had something much worse than ADHD. I was scared of the future – all I saw was bleak, dark times. I worried about Seren as a teenager. If I couldn't cope with her now, what would it be like when her hormones kicked in or when she discovered alcohol or boys ... or both.

As I have said continually, medication is saving lives, but it many instances it is stripping the very thing that we are born with, and that is 'survival'. We have survived as a species for millions of years against all sorts of odds, and yet, now as a society, we are turning to medication to just function in our daily lives.

I have talked before about how Seren got an obsession with death shortly after starting Prozac when she had just turned seven years old. Although the pediatrician had strongly denied that the two were linked, recent press coverage has made me think that I was right in thinking that the medication could have caused this.

Children as young as two are being prescribed antidepressants, which could be leading to higher suicide rates, despite no such medication being recommended for use in children. There are 1,022 Australian children aged 2–6 taking antidepressants, according to the Daily Telegraph. And 26,000 children under the age of sixteen are using the medications.[19]

Many studies have shown a correlation between antidepressant use in children and suicidal ideation, although there is no consensus on the issue in the medical industry. A report released in 2009, by the Therapeutic Goods Administration, found that although SSRI antidepressants (selective serotonin uptake inhibitors) reduced suicide rates among adults, the risk increases among children and adolescents using antidepressants by almost 95%. However, in the four years to 2012–13, the rate of children under the age of sixteen using the drugs rose 42%, according to the Department of Human Services, the Daily Telegraph reported.[19]

And in 2013–14, Australian Institute of Health and Welfare figures showed 95,425 kids under the age of fifteen were using some type of mental health drug.[19]

Hunter-gatherers and farmers

This brings me on to something else that I discovered about ADHD.

I once watched a fantastic interview with Carl 'Thom' Hartmann, who is an American radio host, author, former psychotherapist, entrepreneur and progressive political commentator. He talked about hunter-gatherers and agricultural farmers, and how these could explain the ADHD people of today. The hunter-gatherers needed to be on the go all the time, constantly being aware of predators – so I guess this would explain their 'hyperactivity'. They would have the adrenal surge to fight the predators and they were constantly on the move to make sure that they wouldn't be attacked. He then talked about the farmers who needed to tend to the crops and watch them grow. He said that if you were a hunter-gatherer, you would never be able to stay still and look at the harvest grow. If you were the farmer, you would never be able to fight off the predators. Both personalities were very different; both were needed and so this 'one size fits all' type of education and parenting doesn't suit everyone.[20]

It made complete sense to me (another light bulb moment). But all this aside, none of this was helping me, as I didn't have a damn clue how to parent Seren or how to deal with her violent outbursts, or how to love her. I was lost and it seemed as if medication was my only option!

Medication-free Saturday

We decided that the Ritalin wasn't working and agreed that we wouldn't give Seren the medication on Saturday. However, Seren had a party on Saturday afternoon, which I was worried about. Karl had taken Flynn and Daisy out for the morning and I was going to take Seren to acrobatics and then drop her off at the party.

Seren woke up crazy and was like that all day. We popped out to buy her friend a present and also spend a bit of time together; I thought it might help but it didn't.

I remember losing Seren in the car park and looking for her everywhere. *How could I just lose her, she was right next to me?*

I shouted her name over and over, and walked around for a few minutes wondering where she had gone, before I found her hiding in-between two cars. This should have made me laugh, but at the time, I didn't like Seren (to be honest). Our life was a never-ending nightmare and it was all because of her.

Love/hate

I went from feeling really sorry for her and then hating her, as I couldn't believe we were going through this on a daily basis.

I was sick of the appointments, the meetings, the conversations with friends and family about Seren, and I was tired of talking to Karl about what we could do to 'fix' Seren.

I wasn't aware until much later that during this time my lack of love towards Seren had a terrible effect on her personality and her behaviour. She was so hard to love and even though I did love her – of course I loved her dearly – I was so upset with her that it was hard for me to show her affection.

I didn't realise, at the time, but Seren actually felt that I didn't like her. She felt it from Karl and Daisy, and even Flynn, who would scream when Seren went anywhere near him. He didn't trust her – he had been accidentally dropped or kicked in the head so many times by Seren. Even though Seren loved him desperately, she was so impulsive that being around a baby wasn't always the easiest.

This particular day of the party, I was so angry with Seren, her behaviour was out of control and it continued throughout the day. I had a gut feeling that I shouldn't take her to the party. She was hyper, defiant and out of control, and she was definitely suffering from the 'Ritalin crash'. But she desperately wanted to go to the party. She didn't get invited to play dates or many parties, and she pleaded with me to take her.

I finally agreed to take her, but it turned out to be one of the worst decisions that I have made in my life. However, in hindsight, it was also the turning point for many reasons.

The party

I took Seren to the party and decided to stay and have a chat with some of the mums. It was a sunny autumn day but there was a nip in the air, so the beautiful warm fire burning in a fire pit in the garden was very welcome.

Most of the children were older, around eight or nine, so having the fire pit seemed fine, but to Seren it was a distraction and she couldn't help herself. She danced around it and kept grabbing large handfuls of flowers and throwing them into the fire. She was beyond excitable and was moving very quickly into the 'out of control' phase. Her eyes were wild; her limbs were flailing everywhere and the children and parents were starting to notice that all didn't seem right with Seren.

I tried to ignore it and prayed that she would calm down. I tried to talk to her but she screamed at me, 'Leave me alone, Mum. Go home, just go home'. I stayed an hour in total, chatting to the other mums about kids and life and birthing. I loved talking to them, hearing their views and realising that we all had more in common than I had first realised. I was so happy when one of the mums invited me over for pizza at her house. She said it would be great for our families to get to know each other better. I was talking in depth with them and thoroughly enjoying the conversation; however, at the same time, I kept glancing over at Seren. She was crazy, over the top and extremely hyperactive.

I kept hearing the mum of the party saying, 'Seren, no. Seren, gently. Seren, please don't grab', as she tried in vain to play some party games with the kids.

Again I went over and asked very quietly, 'Seren, please can you calm down, honey. You need to calm down or I will have to stay.'

'Go away, Mum. Shut up, just go.'

Everyone could see how she was speaking to me and I was so embarrassed. All the mums started to leave and I decided that I would go too. Maybe it was me that was making Seren hyper? Maybe the fact that I was there was making her anxious? I was actually looking forward to leaving and having two hours break! Two hours of peace, God I needed it so much – two heavenly hours without Seren, without the craziness, without the drama.

I spoke to the mum of the party and told her that Seren could get a little crazy at parties. 'Sugar can make her go a bit wild, and she gets so excited at parties; please call me if there is a problem.'

'No worries, she will be absolutely fine,' she said. 'They all get a bit excitable at parties.'

I left the house that day feeling a bit worried, but I also had a feeling of freedom, it was wonderful – it washed over me like a warm breeze. We had been in Australia for fifteen months, and we still didn't have any support systems. I desperately needed to sort my life out and get some babysitters. I also dreamt of having a surrogate grandma who could just take Seren for a day, half a day, or even a couple of hours (half an hour would do).

However, this shouldn't have been the day to have some peace and it was probably the worst idea that I have ever had to leave Seren that day. She was out of control, crazy beyond words, and me leaving didn't make her behaviour better, it made her behaviour worse. But at the time of leaving the party, I was so desperate for peace that I did leave, and I wouldn't know the full extent of her behaviour at the party until much later ...

I felt that, although her behaviour was terrible, we had a plan. I had made an appointment to see the pediatrician on the Monday morning and I felt like we were in an elimination process, even though everything was still hard. There had to be a 'safe with little side effects type of drug' for Seren, there just had to be!

The pediatrician had mentioned some other types of medication, one being for epilepsy and this made me feel really happy. Epilepsy is real, I told myself. *My friend has epilepsy and he's ok, he's normal.*

I have since found out that the medication for epilepsy, although life-changing, also comes with massive side effects, which I guess goes back to the concept that 'you can't have your cake and eat it'.

Seren came back from the party and all seemed fine. We shared a bath that night as I felt awful that I had been so unloving to her all day. She was a child with huge issues and I had to stop pushing her aside and being unloving with her. I was her mum; I had to make it right.

We talked about life, and I asked Seren some questions that one of the mums had suggested during our chat at the party. These were questions that you wouldn't usually ask your child, so asking them allowed you to get to know your child a bit better. I had absolutely no idea who Seren was, so this seemed like a great idea!

'What was the first thought you had when you woke up today?'

'What are you most afraid of?'

'What's your favourite word right now and why?'

'What do you love about yourself?'

We continued talking and asking each other questions in the bath – the lights were dimmed, the bath bubbles were overflowing and the candles flickering. It was a moment of serenity and love and I could see how much Seren was enjoying this quality time with me.

Then I asked her, 'Who in your class is lonely?' Without hesitation, she answered, 'Megan'. Megan was a gorgeous little girl in Seren's class who appeared to have ADHD. She also seemed extremely anxious about even coming to school. Every morning when I would drop Seren off at school, Megan would run past me, trying to escape and wanting to be with her mum. I felt for Megan and I felt desperately sad for her mum, as I knew how hard it was to be going through this sort of thing.

Seren didn't suspect that Megan might have ADHD, but she knew something was wrong and she felt very sorry for her.

Correspondence I wrote that weekend – after the party

10 May

Good morning Diane,

Thank you so much for your honesty and your compassion during our meeting on Friday.

Seren won't be coming to school Monday morning as we are going back to see the pediatrician. I will hopefully have Seren back with you for lunchtime.

I am hoping that with the right medication and the continued support from yourself and the other teachers, we can help Seren achieve her true potential.

I had a lovely chat with Seren before bed last night. She talked about how much she loved art and we decided that we would find an art class after school.

Hopefully, all goes well with the pediatrician on Monday.

Kind regards, Susy xx

The party wasn't a success!

After our bath and a lovely Sunday evening together after the craziness on Saturday, I woke up on Monday feeling more positive.

Seren and I shared some breakfast together and then started to get ready to go to the pediatrician. Before leaving the house, the phone rang and it was one of the school mums.

'Hi, how are you?'

'Listen, love, I'm phoning because I care and I'm saying this to help you, to help Seren. I think you need to medicate your child as she I think she has ADHD.'

My heart sank as I listened intently.

The mum then told me how Seren had been extremely wild at the party. Seren had even held her friend's head to the floor while her friend was screaming. She said that all the kids were freaked out and all the mums were really upset. The mum said everyone felt that I let Seren down and that I shouldn't have left her at the party.

I couldn't believe my ears! Seren hadn't mentioned a thing. I felt like we had connected in the bath, how had she not even mentioned all this? Was she scared of telling me or had she simply forgotten?

I told the mum that we thought Seren had ADHD and that she was under a pediatrician. I explained that we had been going through this with Seren for a year and we were very aware that there was a problem.

The mum also told me that all the children were really upset at the party and had to be counselled on the way home. They had never experienced anything like Seren before and now they were all really wary of her.

What the hell had happened at the party? Kids being counselled? Wary of Seren? Was this all a dream? What the hell was going on?

The mum told me that she had first-hand experience with ADHD and that she understood what we were going through. She wanted to offer any support she could.

I hated my life. I felt so out of my depth. I just wanted to go home to the UK and be with my best friends and my family.

I hated all the constant judgement. Of course since then, I have learnt that being judged is something that is going to happen. I have a different type of child, so judgement comes with the territory.

I then called the mum who'd had the party on Saturday. I apologised profusely, but she told me that it had all been blown out of proportion. She said she thought I was a lovely mum and that it must be so hard for us. She was such a caring, nice lady, and as soon as I came off the phone, I bawled my eyes out. I sent her some flowers with a card apologising; it's not every day that your daughter ruins someone's birthday party.

The last call I made was to the mum of Seren's 'best friend'. Seren said this little girl was her 'best friend', but I knew that the feeling wasn't mutual. I'd gone for coffee with this mum a couple of times and we had talked at the party, so I felt awful that Seren had hurt her best friend at the party. This was probably the most difficult conversation that I had with the three mums.

She told me how Seren had forced her daughter's head to the ground and her daughter was now so scared of Seren that she had not been to school that day.

Seren was a lot of things, but a bully? No way! She wouldn't intentionally hurt anyone. She had done lots of things to her brother and sister, and Chip had been thrown off the bunk bed, but it was never intentional, it was only ever impulsive. Her ADHD meant that she didn't think things through before doing them.

This mum said she felt that I had let Seren down as I hadn't stayed at the party with her, and that it would probably be best that we didn't come over for pizza anymore as we had previously planned. I agreed, apologised profusely, said goodbye and then hung up the phone. Lying on the grass outside, I put myself into the foetal position and just cried and cried.

My heart sank; it ached inside. *What was happening? Why was our life, and Seren's behaviour, spiralling out of control? What was going on? But more than anything, why was everyone so fucking mean?*

Correspondence during this time

12 May

Hi Diane,

I learnt yesterday afternoon about what happened at the party, and I've just called the mum and had a long chat with her. I'm just waiting to hear back from the other mums so I can apologise. I have also come to learn about a situation with Seren and one of her friends. Would you like to meet up this week to discuss it? I'm so upset and embarrassed and feel awful for the other parents. Things can only get better from here! I'm hoping anyway.
Love Susy xx

Hi Susy,

Let's catch up this afternoon for a brief talk. I think the principal will contact you soon for a family conference so that we can all help Seren maintain her dignity and self-confidence.
Kind regards,
Diane xx

I went to see Diane, who confirmed that some of the mums had been in to complain, but she had Seren's back and insisted that she wasn't a bully; it was only her impulsiveness that was getting her into trouble. Even Diane believed that Seren was very caring and would give anyone anything.

I recall a time when Diane called me one morning to say that Seren was giving money out to everyone in the class. A note for 10,000 Indonesian rupiah must have seemed like an awful lot to the children, but it was only worth about $1. Seren had been handing the money out like sweets. I joked with the teacher that maybe Seren wanted to be a philanthropist!

Seren would regularly give other children teddies, books, pens, and clothes. She would give anything to anyone and she would make the sweetest cards and pictures for her friends. She desperately wanted to be liked, and while I agreed her behaviour was impulsive and out of control, she wasn't a bully!

Drowning ...

I was drowning. I didn't know what to do anymore. I was convinced that everyone in the school would now know about the party. The story would have been twisted and changed several times, and people would make assumptions about out family, about Karl, about me.

Diary entries and correspondence during this time

13 May

Seren seemed very agitated tonight. She slept with me and was still wide-awake at 12.00 am; she said her heartbeat was keeping her awake. She made me so sad and also so worried. The very first pediatrician we saw stated that Seren had a heart murmur so this worries me as the second pediatrician didn't do any tests. I managed to give her some lavender and then she calmed down. I hugged her to sleep. I spoke to the mums again at school and I made an appointment to see Diane, Seren's teacher.

14 May

Seren seems very agitated at home, her hands and face are clammy, her heart racing. She cries and says that she feels worse, she feels scared. She feels everyone is talking about her and she has been very impulsive at school. I saw her sweeping up at school today and she seemed hyper and defiant with the other children.

Her teachers said she is ok in the morning, but by the time she has the second dose, she seems detached. She is nasty to the children with unkind words but then is unaware that she has said these words.

Her writing has become very small and is now so hard to read. She seems zoned out at night and she is only able to watch TV. She screams when it's switched off before dinner and has a screaming tantrum on the floor like a toddler.

I am giving her so much love and remained calm. Putting her to bed was a nightmare, Karl and I tried and it took over an hour. She ended up sleeping under the bed. The only medication that seemed to work for Seren was a mood stabiliser. I am quite convinced that Seren's biggest problem is not ADHD but something else.

I am thinking that all the medication should be stopped (other than the Prozac) until we know what we are dealing with. When I give Seren an instruction, she glares at me in a very unnerving way. She seems to look through me. Since we have stopped the Risperidone, Seren has not been able to do any tasks at home. She used to do all her jobs, help me around the house and get herself ready. She is now unable to do anything. :-(

15 May

I met with Seren's teacher and the principal of the school. A lot of the mums from the party have been to see the teacher and the principal to complain about Seren.

The principal supports us and our journey with Seren. She said she understood what we were going through and that she would be there for us. She went on to say that Seren was a beautiful little girl who would hug her every time she saw her. I found myself crying through most of the meeting. What's happening to me? I am falling apart.

I have also booked Seren to see a doctor that the principal recommended. I have been told that he is quite the maverick and is very different in his approach, but she said he was fantastic.

I'm going to find a psychiatrist to work with Seren now too, as I am convinced something else is happening.

Diane agrees that the mood stabiliser was the best type of medication for Seren – Seren was happy, calm and able to do her work.

She seemed great at home today, only becoming defiant and hyper when the routine changed. I've got to massively step up my loving and my parenting now and help this little girl!

15 May

Hi Diane,

The pediatrician is off today and Monday, but I feel that it's probably best to not give Seren the lunchtime medication. I've booked a meeting with the doctor that the principal recommended on Monday at 2.30 pm, so if it's ok with you I will collect Seren at 2.00 pm.

Seren will have to undergo lots of tests and examinations beforehand, which I believe will be done on Monday. Once all the results are through, we will then meet with the doctor again.

I'm also going to get Seren seen by a psychiatrist too, as I'm afraid that there is something we might be missing.

I hope she is ok today.

Thank you as always for your continued support.

Have a great weekend!

Lots of love, Susy xx

Hi Susy,

Wow! You really are onto it. Well done!

We will not give her the lunch dose and see if that changes her pm behaviour.

She is loud and a little agitated, but no problem.

She did lots of work and was proud of herself and very apologetic if she did something wrong or we asked her to be quiet.

I will see how her sports teacher found her at sport when they return. Take care.

Diane xx

16 May

I found out today that Seren had been stealing from acrobatics. :-(She was very hyper and defiant today.

17 May

We went to friends for dinner. Seren was out of control. Her hyperactivity levels are now ridiculous. She stole money out of her friend's money jar and all hell broke loose. That night she pretended to be scared of me again. She went to bed crying and pretending to shake and be frightened of me even though I was very calm and loving.

18 May

I have found out that Seren could either be on the autism spectrum disorder or she could be ADHD Type Six? Going to send her to both the counsellor and the pediatrician. I am thinking that the pediatrician will prescribe Seren with a mood stabiliser. This coupled with counselling sessions and a session with the psychiatrist, and continued support from the school should help.

When she's settled I would like to get her back into swimming lessons, playing an instrument or dancing, something to try and channel her behaviour in a different direction.

18 May

Hi Susy,

It has been very difficult with Seren today. She needs to work alone because her interactions with her peers have been disruptive and erratic. This will calm her down and help her control herself. She has her own table and I will monitor her work in a positive and encouraging way!

Diane xx

Hi Diane,

Oh dear, I did suspect this. We have been having a very difficult time with her too, and we are at a loss as to how to manage her behaviour. I've got an appointment with the pediatrician on Wednesday, but I'm not going to take Seren with me, there are things I need to discuss with him that I can't discuss in front of her. Karl will come with me too, as he usually doesn't attend the appointments.

The counsellor thinks as I do that it's time to see a psychiatrist, as I'm really unsure with the ADHD/ODD diagnosis – there could be something that we are missing? I'm also going to ask the pediatrician to refer Seren to a neurologist, as I've been told this will help us to identify what is going on with her.

My mum, Karen, and a friend both asked me to look into Pathological Demand Avoidance Syndrome. There is a link below and I would be so grateful if you would have a quick look and let me know if you feel Seren displays this sort of behaviour in school.

We feel it pretty much sums Seren up; I just wanted to know your thoughts on it.

Thank you so much, Diane.
Susy xx

Hi Susy,

Yes, I agree, many of these attributes fit with her behaviour. I guess the root of her behaviour is impulsiveness, which is not talked about here in this article. The thing is she doesn't avoid doing things at school – she just gets side-tracked doing them when other people cross her path, and then she wants to help, advise, control, organise them instead! How she does this lacks social cues and empathy, which puts her in a poor social interaction state.

Diane xx

Hi Diane,

I see what you mean – maybe it's not that? I have also been advised that there are six types of ADHD, and stimulants only work for a few of them. I'm pretty sure Seren is a ring of fire (God help me), and this can be determined by the neurologist and the outcome of brain scans. I feel this also describes Seren, what do you think? I hope you don't mind me asking you. I will leave it in the capable hands of the experts; I'm just interested in your thoughts.

Thank you, Diane!
Love Susy xx

Letter to the pediatrician

19 May

I am coming to see you today so I will give you an update when I arrive. The second lot of medication didn't work either and this was also confirmed by Seren's teacher on Friday. There were various reasons why it didn't work and I can discuss these with you when I see you. I do remember some time ago you felt that stimulants would make Seren's defiant behaviour worse, and you were right.

I have come across a couple of things since we last met, and I would like to bring both of them to your attention and would welcome your thoughts.

I am also convinced that Seren is ADHD Type Six. I have been told that a brain scan with a neurologist could determine the type of ADHD Seren has – would you be able to write me a referral letter to a child neurologist, please?

I also want to talk to you about Pathological Avoidance Syndrome, which is on the autistic spectrum.

Looking forward to meeting with you later.

Kind regards, Susy.

Rock bottom ...

I had officially hit rock bottom; although, it felt much worse than rock bottom, it felt like hell. I had gone as far as I could go with the pediatrician – he had offered me Seroquel for Seren, a potent antipsychotic drug.

A condemning report published by CBC News in 2014, highlighted that Seroquel (and I quote) 'A powerful mood-altering medication with potentially life-threatening side effects was for years being prescribed in Canadian prisons for unapproved purposes, raising concerns the drug was being used to "subdue" or "sedate" inmates', a joint CBC News/Canadian Press investigation has revealed.[21]

It's interesting that they are alarmed that this drug is being used incorrectly on prisoners, yet here in Perth, it's completely fine to give it to a seven- year-old girl! Even the handout that the pediatrician gave me stated that Seroquel should not be used in children under fourteen, and here I was with a prescription for this medication for my seven-year-old daughter.

Seroquel is a strong sedative used to treat bipolar and schizophrenia but the pediatrician had confirmed that Seren didn't have either of these conditions. This new medication made Risperidone look like candy floss! The side effects of taking Seroquel were hyperglycaemia, high blood pressure and diabetes, and these are some of the nicer side effects – believe me, there are many, many more.

This had to stop! This was getting out of hand. How could I give such a strong drug to my seven-year-old child? How could this be acceptable? I knew things had to change and I knew I was the only one that could make a difference. I couldn't let this continue. I had to get a hold on my fucking life, on Seren's life!

But I didn't know where to start? I couldn't breathe. I couldn't think straight. I was desperately lonely, isolated and at the end.

Plan for Seren

23 May
- Sound therapy
- Psychologist
- Essential oils
- Pediatrician
- Hope and pray
- Calm parenting
- Loving home
- CAMHS
- Support meetings.

Time without her

Karl could see what it was doing to me, so he suggested taking Seren away for the weekend. He felt that his relationship with Seren was non-existent, so he wanted to take her away for the weekend so they could spend some time together. He wanted to give me some breathing space, but I was scared to be on my own. However, at the same time, I knew it would be perfect for Seren.

Karl left that Friday night with a very excited Seren, and as soon as he left the anxiety I felt kicked in. He told me to relax and take it easy, just enjoy Daisy and Flynn, but I knew that all I would end up doing was more research.

I had to find another way. I just had to! There was no other option. I could not fail. I could not let Seren down. I couldn't let myself and my beautiful family down anymore.

I suddenly felt like Neo in The Matrix film, and before me stood Morpheus saying, 'You take the blue pill, the story ends. You wake up in your bed and believe whatever you want to believe. You take the red pill, you stay in wonderland, and I show you how deep the rabbit hole goes'.

I could have taken the blue pill (metaphorically speaking), which would have meant doing what the pediatrician suggested, the psychologist suggested, and the teachers suggested. Everything would be so much easier for everyone if I just did as I was told – medicate my out of control child – but where would that have left Seren? What would it do to her in the long run?

So I took the red pill (metaphorically speaking), and as soon as I did, things started to change for the better.

More support

That weekend of 'freedom', I talked to one of my oldest friends in the UK. Mandy had been a friend of mine for twenty-five years. She wasn't a friend that I spoke to very often, but we had a deep love and appreciation for each other. Anna had told Mandy what was going on with Seren and, as Mandy had just qualified as a health visitor in the UK, she had a keen interest in what was happening with Seren.

I chatted on the phone with Mandy for nearly two hours. She listened, she gave advice and, in a way, she saved me before I totally lost myself. She said something to me that will stay with me always. 'Mums are the glue of the family. They keep everything together. How can you keep everything together when you are falling apart yourself, Susy?'

She told me that in France, they don't have a big problem with ADHD as they deal with it from a 'whole family approach' that looks at interactions between parents and siblings. They help the family and the school to learn how to cope with ADHD and how to strengthen the bond and the family unit, without medication. Medication can sometimes just be a bandaid. Once you stop the medication, the behaviour returns. And in our case, the medication was causing Seren's behaviour to become worse. She said that while the UK did medicate, the health visitors would work with the family, looking at parenting, diet etc.

I had so wanted to have that here in Australia, instead of just being exposed to the 'take this pill and everything will be ok' approach. It wasn't ok – her behaviour was better, but with that came a whole heap of disturbing side effects. Side effects that over time could become even worse than Seren's poor childhood behaviour – these side effects could change everything forever.

Mandy talked about how she wasn't an advocate for stimulant medication in children, but she did say how she felt medication would help me. She advised me to go to the doctors and ask for a low-dose antidepressant for myself, and she recommended Sertraline. I was so scared, I had never taken anything in my life, but I knew she was right.

I was spiralling down further and further into darkness and I couldn't seem to do anything about it.

Heading back to the UK

We were leaving Australia and travelling back to the UK for Karl's sister's wedding in just four weeks. I was in complete panic mode, and all I had were black, dark thoughts:

Seren's behaviour would be out of control.

We had a long-haul flight.

We had to face everyone, and friends and family would know about Seren.

I had to be happy as a matron of honour, organise a hen do, family and friends get-togethers.

What if it made me really homesick and I didn't want to come back to Australia?

I cried all day, every day, I was a mess and I knew it.

I wrote this in my diary to read to my GP as I knew the minute I stepped into his office, I would be as bright as a button – I was so good at faking it!

25 May

I'm having a very stressful time with my eldest daughter who has ADHD and ODD. It's a continuously changing situation that is getting better in some ways but not in others, and I am finding it's taking a huge chunk of my daily thoughts. I'm also quite convinced that I too have ADHD.

I have been stressed and depressed for most of my life. I suffer from mood swings that are particularly extreme around ovulation and my period, which cause me to honestly think that being dead would be better off (although I would never want to leave my children, so I go off this idea very quickly). I hate myself, feel ugly, hate my figure, hate my skin. I try and tell myself over and over of all the things that I need to be grateful for but that doesn't stop the self-loathing.

For parts of the month I am happy, truly happy and at peace, but most of the time I'm stressed, worried and anxious! My thoughts race continually and I'm never at peace. I've always slept well but now I don't, so I'm also exhausted. I exercise 3–4 times per week. I eat well, drink little coffee, and devote my life to my children.

No-one would ever know that I feel like this other than my husband. All my friends and family say I'm such a positive person, yet I'm dying inside. I practice yoga, meditation (ok only once a week) … I try all sorts of positivity through rocks, crystals, oils etc. but they are only short-lived. I have honestly thought that I probably need to be on antidepressants and I have felt like this for about seven years!

What shall I do?

Love Susy xx

I need drugs!

I chickened out and didn't read the message to him, but I did tell him that I felt like I needed antidepressants.

He didn't agree. 'You are not depressed, Susy, you are just trying to cope with a very stressful situation away from all your family and friends.'

'No really, I am depressed. I am anxious. I am not coping, please can I have some Sertraline?' I replied.

'Why don't you go and see the naturopath and see if she has got something for you?'

I couldn't believe that I had a pantry full of drugs for my seven-year-old that would rival the local drug dealer, but I couldn't get any antidepressants for myself. I am actually very thankful to my doctor, he made me feel very normal and I did come to understand that there was nothing wrong me.

On a separate note, though, since I had Flynn, I had struggled with my moods around ovulation and during my period. I would get down, emotional and angry. I would start self-loathing and not being very nice to Karl. Then the clouds would go away and I would be fine again. I would happy, madly in love with Karl again, and everything would be fine in 'Susy World', but then it would change again.

What a roller coaster! I also found Seren almost impossible to deal with when I felt like this. I don't really remember writing that note to my doctor, and I don't ever remember feeling that bad, maybe I was depressed after all? I certainly felt like I was, and I don't feel like that anymore, so I am very glad that he did actually prescribe me the Sertraline, although he said he would only give me a two-month prescription.

I decided only to take a quarter of the recommended dose, which meant that I was on just 12.5 mg. It made me feel better instantly and it helped me through a very dark period in my life. So, here I was, now medicating myself after having been so dead-set against medication ...

I honestly feel that medication has a place in society and I am thankful that it helped me. I stayed on the medication for just a few months and then took myself off it. It had served its purpose and helped me through a very difficult time. While on it, I was able to see clearly, make decisions, and stay focused while helping my daughter.

Daisy's birthday party was coming up, and before I took the medication I couldn't even think about. But when I was on the medication, I was excitedly planning her party, along with the trip to the UK, and everything else for that matter!

I stopped crying and that dark, bloody cloud that had been stalking me for the last few months suddenly disappeared.

Going against the suggestion – letter to the pediatrician

22 May

Thank you so much as always for your time this week. I have decided that I'm not at the point where I can give antipsychotic medicine to Seren. For me this has to be the last option.

I have spoken to the Complex Attention and Hyperactivity Disorders Service today and they will see Seren, but they need a referral letter from you. I would be so grateful if you would write a referral letter to them. They have a team there who will work with both our family and the school, which I feel Seren needs right now.

I'm very thankful for the help you have given me so far.

Kind regards, Susy

I think it might be pretty obvious how I really felt about the peditrician. The first letter didn't read anything like that. I never intended to send him that first one; I just needed to get it off my chest. We were also right in the middle of a desperately hard time with Seren, and I didn't know whether I would ever have to go and see the pediatrician again. Keep your own counsel, I told myself, make the right choice. Be dignified.

Desperate for a team

I decided to watch the UK TV program, *Born Naughty* again.

The little girl did have some similarities to Seren. It was fascinating as, just like us, the parents were gentle and calm, yet the girl's reaction was as if they were monsters trying to attack her. She screamed and yelled and ran out of the house. She fought with them, spat at them and had just been expelled from school.

Seren's behaviour, although not as bad as that, was getting out of control.

She was hiding in the toilets now at school and was also trying to escape from school on a daily basis.

A team of people assessed the girl on the TV show – there was a pediatrician, a psychologist, a psychiatrist, and a speech pathologist. The little girl was assessed over some weeks at home and in the clinic. I thought that this was exactly what I needed for Seren.

Although our counsellor had reassured me that she would do this, I had tried in vain to get back in touch with her but she hadn't contacted me back. She had suggested that Seren might need to see a psychiatrist but that the good ones had closed their books. At best, I could be looking at a waiting time of twelve months.

Closed their books? This was one of the scariest things that I had ever heard! *What is wrong with all the children here in Perth? What is going wrong?*

I remember phoning the counsellor; the rain was beating down so hard that day that I could barely hear what she was saying on the phone. She promised she would try and find a psychiatrist or another pediatrician, but sadly she never did. I sent her Diane's details too, but she never got in contact with Diane either.

In a way I am happy that she didn't get back to me. She gave me some great information and put me on a new path, so I will be eternally grateful for that.

Another wonderful babysitter

During this time we had a beautiful French babysitter called Rosie, she would occasionally babysit for us at night when Karl and I would go out on a date. She was in her 50s and Seren adored her. Karl and I hadn't been out for ages and it had been some months since we had seen Rosie, so she was really shocked to see how bad Seren had become.

After babysitting the children that night, Rosie called me the very next day. She told me how Seren had cried to her and said, 'Mummy doesn't love me. Mummy thinks I am naughty. Everyone thinks I am naughty. I am not like other people'. Rosie told me that she said to Seren, 'Mummy loves you very much. She only wants the best for you'.

Rosie went on to say to me that her husband used to be a doctor and he always told her, 'Don't go and see a psychiatrist, they will make you mad. They make things up that aren't there'.

Although I know this isn't the absolute truth about psychiatrists, it was a comment that stayed with me nonetheless, and I am so thankful that she had called me that day.

The little girl on the TV show was eventually diagnosed with Pathological Avoidance Syndrome, which is part of the autistic spectrum. I was quite convinced that Seren had it – when Karl and I read out all the symptoms, it was like it was written for Seren.

The centre that the little girl had gone to was in Nottingham in the UK, and we were going to the UK in four weeks!

This was it. This was the answer! If we couldn't get any help here in Perth, we could get some help when we got to the UK!

I called them, but they were closed in July. I needed to try and find somewhere like this in Perth. In sheer desperation, I posted this message to a Facebook group.

Message to Poms in Perth Facebook group

24 May

Hi everyone, we've been here for sixteen months and everything was great until we started having some very serious behavioural problems with our eldest daughter. She is nearly eight and I'm finding here that all they want to do is diagnose her with ADHD and give her strong antipsychotic drugs. We've spent $1000s of dollars on pediatricians, psychologists, naturopaths, and the problem is worse than ever. I am struggling to find support here. I spoke to my friend in the UK last night who is a health visitor and she said that there is so much support in the UK for this, support for families and from the school. I'm now thinking of moving back to the UK, to get the support of friends and family who we all miss so much. I dread the move back but just wondered if anyone had gone through a similar thing and moved back home. I love it here will all my heart, but it seems that the specialists here are stuck in the dark ages when it comes to mental health.

Thanks for your advice in advance.

What was so lovely was that I had over seventy different messages with support and guidance. Many people said that they had wonderful support here, and many said that the UK was better. It seemed to be completely split, and it appeared that the UK had its problems too.

We loved living in Australia. We loved everything about it and I felt so lucky and grateful to live here and to raise my children here, but I was outraged at what was being allowed and deemed acceptable to do to children.

CAHDS

A few people told me about a service here in Perth called Complex Attention and Hyperactivity Disorder Service (CAHDS). It was a free service and it was exactly what I was looking for. A team of experts would assess Seren, and then they would make the assessment after six weeks.

It had to be done through the pediatrician, as CAHDS would send the report back to them. So I emailed the pediatrician and I also spoke to my own GP about this group. I was surprised that neither of them had ever heard of this service, yet it was a government service and was part of the Child and Adolescent Mental Health Service (CAMHS).

How could nobody know about this and why wasn't Seren assessed in this way before being prescribed a cocktail of drugs?

Just to confirm, Seren had been prescribed the following medications:

- Fluoxteine (Prozac) – used for depression and anxiety
- Ritalin – used for ADHD
- Dextroamphetamine – used for ADHD
- Risperidone – used for bipolar and schizophrenia
- Seroquel – used for bipolar and schizophrenia

I find it so hard to believe that a child can be prescribed all of these medications in such a small amount of time, without this kind of proper testing and monitoring. There was no testing at home or school. The school and Karl and I had completed a Connors test, but Seren had been medicated with both Ritalin and Prozac before the test had even been done.

And how is the test even accurate? One little questionnaire and then just like that – medication!

Interestingly, Keith Conners, a psychologist and early advocate for recognition of ADHD, addressed a group of fellow ADHD specialists in Washington in 2013. He noted that recent data from the Centers for Disease Control and Prevention show that the diagnosis had been made in 15% of high school-aged children, and that the number of children on medication for the disorder had soared to 3.5 million from 600,000 in 1990. He questioned the rising rates of diagnosis and called them 'a national disaster of dangerous proportions'. 'The numbers make it look like an epidemic. Well, it's not. It's preposterous,' he said in a subsequent interview. 'This is a concoction to justify the giving out of medication at unprecedented and unjustifiable levels.'[22]

Now what does that tell us?

Chapter Nine

Tests, tests and more tests just for good measure

The phlebotomist at the pathology centre said that she had never taken so many samples of blood from one person. I think I remember there being twenty-one! Twenty-one little bottles of Seren's blood all sat in a tray. Was her blood the key to the many questions we had? Only time would tell ...

Our appointment date arrived to see the 'new' doctor recommended to me by the school principal. He was a bit alternative, but he was the first person who made me realise, or believe, that ADHD wasn't a disorder or an illness, it was just Seren's personality.

First meeting with the new doctor

We met with the 'researcher' first and she asked us hundreds of questions, mostly these questions were linked to adults and people with obesity and major health problems. Various tests were done, such as heart rate, pulse rates etc., and then the doctor popped in for a chat.

Seren was her usual crazy self – jumping up and down on the examination bed and pressing the button so the bed went up and down and then up and down again.

The doctor was very cool. I remember he had a very unusual bedside manner as well as rather outlandish shoes. He immediately said to Seren,

'Did you not the see the sign on the way in, it said "no children". I don't like children', and with this Seren fell about laughing. He was as mad as her and she loved him!

He told me that she was living off her adrenaline and that giving her a stimulant would only make that worse. He wasn't a fan of the 'ADHD Club' and he believed that other factors needed to be looked into first. He said that we would both need to go for some blood tests and then we would need to come back and see him in a couple of weeks.

He also suggested giving Seren some glucose from the chemist after school, or when she started to get very hyperactive. It felt nice going to the chemist that night and asking for 'glucose' instead of handing over a prescription. Oh, and just to point out, I tried the glucose but it had very little effect!

More blood tests, results and suggestions

After much cajoling and bribing, I managed to get Seren to go for a blood test. Seren went first and then I went after her. She was so brave and the nurses were lovely with her.

Yet again the ADHD kicked in and Seren touched and played with everything in the pathologist's office. And again, Seren found the examination bed button and was kindly told by the lady, numerous times, to stop. Of course, Seren ignored her and the bed went up and down and up and down ...

Nothing was easy with little Seren – every appointment, every meeting was hard. Seren always has, and still does, need to touch everything and anything. It used to drive me insane, but now I just accept it; it's what she does, it's how she feels, it's what drives her. I now don't say 'don't touch', as there is very little point – she simply has to touch and feel things.

The results came back from the blood tests and Seren and I went back to the doctor. Seren had hated going to all the appointments, and she would mostly cower every time we would go, which was horrible, but she was very excited about going back to see this doctor. 'He's really funny, Mummy. I like him.' This was happy news to me.

The doctor was a highly intelligent man, who often spoke in riddles and it was very hard to understand him at times, but the consensus was that Seren was pretty much low in everything! Iron, vitamin B, vitamin D, iodine, the list was endless!

He also said that she had low blood flow to the gut and therefore she wasn't able to absorb iron and other such things, which he felt was a contributing factor to her behaviour. He also stated that she was on a high dose of Prozac and that we needed to change this straightaway. Seren was on 20 mg of Prozac, so the doctor suggested that we changed it to 5 mg; he felt that this would be better for her.

He then told me how he disagreed with all the pediatricians and the pharmaceutical companies. He felt that we were just 'dumbing down' these highly intelligent, different kids. He told me how special Seren was and that I needed a medal for the last seven years!

He was slightly mad, but I loved him as he was so eccentric and different and I was fed up with the 'one size fits all' medical system. Throughout the meeting he made calls and answered his phone numerous times. I had never come across a professional like him, but I loved his ideas and they made sense.

He told me, 'We have got no more fucking Einsteins, no great inventors anymore'; 'They don't want people to think outside the box, they want to just fucking dumb them down, medicate them, let them all think and learn the same'; 'Don't do it to Seren, don't let them do it to her'; 'She is special, she will be great; you will see'.

He then suggested that we go for a walk. We left the surgery, walking past his patients in the waiting room (who I suspect had also been waiting for him for the previous two hours).

We walked and talked for about thirty minutes and he taught Seren about cloud formations. It was one of the strangest appointments I have had, but Seren loved it!

'Look at her, she's not attention deficit, she is just different,' he said.

He and Seren had more in common than I realised, and if anyone had ADHD, I think it was this doctor, but he had a brilliant mind that definitely 'thought outside the box'.

I went on to tell the doctor that I was taking Sertraline. I said that I felt great and that it started working straightaway. He told me that I wasn't depressed as there was no way that the drug could start to work straightaway. He told me that it was just giving me more blood flow to the brain and that the 5 mg of Prozac would essentially do the same to Seren, without all the side effects.

He said that I only needed to take a very small amount of the Sertraline, and that I would never need the full dosage. He also wanted to send Seren for a brain scan. Following on from the scan, he would then be able to medicate her, but it wouldn't be a stimulant, it would be a very different type of drug with few side effects.

We left that day not quite sure about what had just happened; however, I somehow felt relieved. I had written down everything he said, and vowed to implement the changes when we got home.

We were now using 'Magic 1,2,3', and the money in the jar, which was going well. There were fewer time-outs, less shouting and much more love.

Another wonderful babysitter – with ADHD

During this more recent time, I managed to find a babysitter called Jade. She was twenty-four and was studying to be a marine biologist. She also had ADHD, so had lots of experience with it!

I found her on a carers Facebook group and she came into our lives at just the right time. We desperately needed some respite, so a couple of times a month, Jade would take Seren out for a few hours at the weekend.

Seren adored Jade (she was like a grown-up version of Seren), excitable, talkative, loved bike rides, craft, art, climbing trees, all the things that Seren loved. It also gave me a great bargaining tool to help with Seren's behaviour as Jade became the reward – genius!

Iron infusion

As Seren and I were very low in iron, the doctor arranged for us to have an iron infusion. Again I popped off to the chemist to pick up the prescription for Ferinject. Apparently this isn't supposed to be used for children under fourteen, and trying to get a doctor to do this (other than ours), can be difficult.

But Seroquel on the other hand, which is used in prisons to sedate inmates, seems to be fine! Anyway, thank God I wasn't giving her Seroquel, so I happily skipped to the chemist to pick up friendly, happy, non-powerful mood-altering phials of Ferinject.

I collected two phials of Ferinject and, using my 'bribery Jade tactics' and a fluffy toy dog that we had seen at the chemist, Seren had her iron infusion.

It took about ten minutes and felt 'a bit funny' according to Seren, but never the less she did it, as did I, and then we went off to buy the fluffy dog.

The doctor had told us that it would take about 2–3 weeks to notice a difference, and I worked out we would be in the UK when it came into effect, and so I arranged for the brain scan for when we got back. However, only days after Seren had the infusion, we noticed that her tic had gone! Just like that, she stopped moving her head up and down, and her limbs stopped flying around everywhere – this was the start of many more miracles to come.

Things on the up!

Seren was now taking taurine, fluoxetine, folonic acid, thiamine, Creon and fludrocortisone under our new doctor. Most of these medications were natural, other than the fluoxetine and fludrocortisone.

He had reduced the fluoxetine (Prozac) from 20 mg to just 5 mg, and although I knew very little about fludrocortisone, it wasn't as bad as Risperidone or Seroquel, so I felt at peace with my decision.

Things for the first time in a long while seemed to be on the up. I was finally crawling out from the rock bottom home that I had been mentally living in for the last number of months.

We also decided that we would start using essential oils on her. This was my way of saying goodbye once and for all to the medication route for Seren. From now on, it was going to be natural all the way (although I was soon to realise that some of the medication prescribed by our new doctor wasn't as natural as I first thought)!

Diary entries during this time

7 June
Methods that are working:
- 'Magic 1,2,3'
- Money in the jar
- Jade (giving us some respite)
- School being more loving and caring
- Me being calm and loving
- New doctor – getting blood tests on Tuesday, may start medication.

I've been on antidepressants (only a very low dose now) for eight days. I am so much calmer and happier and so is Seren! Could this be linked? Interesting?

When we get home from the UK, we have an appointment with CAHDS. I am hoping that as soon as we know what's going on with little Seren, we will know how to proceed! All in all it's going well!!!!!! :-) Thank you.

24 June

Seren's behaviour has been a lot better; she has been less defiant and easier to manage. However, her impulsivity and hyperactivity are no different. She can concentrate better in school but she is still unable to make friends and is difficult to manage.

She is now taking medication from the pediatrician. She has had intro-iron, which should kick in – in three weeks.

The doctor said to make sure her diet is good. She was so difficult last night at the dinner for Daisy's birthday. She was out of control! Next time we need to take the iPad as the craft just isn't cutting it! She needs to be told 'no ice-cream if your behaviour is bad'. She has to learn!

29 June

Seren's behaviour is great! Jade is helping so much. She does get hyper but only when she is tired or at the end of her school day. I can handle it better now, as before I honestly couldn't cope. Seren does seem better, only getting hyper when we are out or when a lot is happening.

Overall her behaviour is so much better and I am really happy that it's going in the right direction.

The UK trip

The UK trip came and went and I was glad that due to the abysmal weather, all my homesickness went and I couldn't wait to get back to Australia. It was wonderful spending time with family and friends and, besides a couple of incidents, Seren's behaviour was amazing.

However, I knew that this would change as soon as we arrived back in Australia, as Seren didn't cope well with change. Once again she would have to say goodbye to all our family and friends.

Back in Australia

The day after we arrived back in Australia, Karl was going snowboarding with his friend. I knew Seren wouldn't cope very well with this and I was so worried about Karl going away. In fact, I was dreading it.

The very next day after Karl left, Seren's behaviour took another massive nosedive.

Karl had gone away with his friend, Pete, who also had ADHD. Pete always told us how he was diagnosed in the 70s with ADHD, although then it was called 'hyperactivity'. He said his dad was very strict but his mum and grandmother gave him so much affection. He told us that despite all the negativity that he endured from teachers, family and friends, to him 'it was just like water off a duck's back', as his mum and grandmother showered him with love.

He had never been medicated and at forty-seven years of age, he was married to a great woman and they had two beautiful kids. He was intelligent, witty, successful, an entrepreneur, and talked a million miles an hour.

Pete's wife Marie and their two daughters came to stay the night with us while the boys were away. It was during this time that Marie witnessed Seren's hyperactive, out of control and defiant behaviour. Marie was astounded by it. Seren wouldn't respond to a simple instruction and it was so hard to remain calm, even though 'remaining calm' had now become my new middle name!

Marie praised me on my ability to not 'lose my cool'. I told her over a glass or two or three of wine that night what we had been through over the last year. In fact, it was incredible to let go of a lot of stuff that I had been harbouring. I was finally getting things off my chest. We talked for hours and I realised that I was very lucky as I just found a really good friend, someone who 'got it' as her husband also had ADHD.

Diary entry during this time

31 July
What has happened with our daughter is nothing short of amazing! It will be so interesting to see how Seren gets on at school on Monday. Yes, she is still cheeky, defiant and rude, but she is only seven and she is my daughter. I have been on Sertraline now for two months and

the difference in me is amazing, a lot of it I am sure is down to Seren's behaviour.

I can cope with everything much better, and parent Seren better. It's a miracle! Seren is never going to be an easy kid, she's feisty, quirky and says stuff before she thinks, but she has a heart of gold and is a kind, caring little girl. I wasn't able to see any of this before, as she was so bad and I was so depressed. She has been on the medication with the doctor for the last six weeks and she is so much better.

The plan with our new doctor

The plan was simple – take the various medications he'd prescribed for a month while we were in the UK, then come back and have the brain scan and then we would go from there.

The brain scan might sound odd, but I had been reading lots of information all about the different types of ADHD and how different medication worked for different children.

I had also come across someone whose child had had the brain scan and it had identified which type of ADHD he was and which medication would be better for him.

Days after landing home, I tried to contact our doctor; however, all his numbers were disconnected. I couldn't understand it, where had he gone?

I called the chemist where we had got the prescription from as we had run out of everything. The chemist gave me an email address, so I contacted the doctor and hoped for the best.

No more doctor!

The doctor eventually came back to me and told me that at the moment he wasn't practising.

I emailed him back and said how sorry I was, but pleaded with him to help us and at least write another prescription. Unfortunately, he never got back to me. I felt sorry for his situation but I was very cross that he had written the prescriptions, which we had used, and now we were left in the lurch.

I went to see my GP to see if he could write the prescription, but he said, 'Susy, I am sorry, I do not agree with the prescription and I cannot give you a repeat for this, no-one will. It just doesn't make sense why he had prescribed all this'.

That was it, just like that. The end of the line ... again.

Diary entry during this time

8 August

We came home and Seren's difficult behaviour started, in fact it started two days before we left the UK. I felt it was due to the: 'there'll soon be change'. We came back to Oz and then Daddy left for snowboarding. Seren's behaviour started to get out of control again! :-(

The doctor isn't practising anymore and I can no longer get hold of him or get a repeat prescription and we have now run out of some of the medication that he prescribed – honestly, you couldn't make this shit up! I am still thinking of continuing with the folonic acid, thiamine and taurine, as these are natural. We have gone back to the essential oils and they have been amazing! I am trying to cut out dairy and gluten again too.

Seren's behaviour has been outstanding since we started on the oils again. I have been love-bombing her lots and lots! :-)

Thinking of sharing my story – Seren's story to help other children.

Karl's accident

Karl was on day three of snowboarding when he had a freak accident. Karl's passion, other than surfing, motorbikes and cars, was most definitely snowboarding. He went twice a year, every year, and was a very experienced rider. However, on this holiday he accidentally tripped and fell on his friend's snowboard.

Karl thought he was fine but Pete saw the blood, then the injury, and then covered Karl's eyes. Karl was taken down the mountain on a stretcher (something that to this day he thinks is worse than his injury as it's so embarrassing).

He had cut right through two tendons – his patella tendon and his ITB tendon. He was taken immediately to hospital and given three levels of stitches as the surgeon had to sew the tendon back together, then the muscle and finally the skin. Karl was shaken up but he was ok. It could have been much worse.

One of the side effects for me with the antidepressants was that I was unable to cry. I would sometimes feel it about to come, and get quite excited about the prospect of having a weep, but then in a flash it would be gone, just like that, and us girls do like a little cry now and again.

Even though I was so worried and upset about Karl, I couldn't cry. In a way I had become like my grandmother, I had finally grown some big shoulders and become stoic! I would dig deep, stand tall and get on with it all.

Karl came home bruised and battered, with a cast, and with some attractive crutches. He couldn't walk, and was quite unable to do anything. The surgeon had told him that he was not to move his leg and that he had to keep it straight at all times, take his painkillers and rest. Karl was unable to move from the sofa other than the odd highlight of the day that involved going to the toilet!

Seren's behaviour now had worsened and I was not only trying to keep myself calm for Seren, but I had also turned into a single mother and a carer for my husband! I have so much respect for single mums and dads – it's a bloody tough job trying to do everything.

The days passed, Karl went to different doctors appointments, and I started to get into this new way of life.

Little did I know that life was about to turn on its head completely and bring our lives crashing down once again!

Chapter Ten

When your life flashes before you, suddenly everything makes sense (well sort of)

They say you don't know what you've got until it's gone. The truth is, you knew what you had. You just never thought that you'd lose it. To think what could have happened, what I could have lost ... it didn't even bear thinking about.

It was 20th August – I got the kids to bed, tidied up and then went to bed myself. I was absolutely exhausted, the children were sick with the flu and I had also caught it. I had a cough that was so bad my chest wheezed, my nose ran, and I ached all over.

With poorly kids and a poorly husband, our family sleeping arrangements had gone to shit, and every night someone was sleeping somewhere different.

Karl slept on the sofa. Seren now slept in our bed with Daisy, and I had started sleeping upstairs in the spare room. The only person who slept in his own bed was Flynn!

Now Karl's really sick ...

This particular night, Daisy had wanted to sleep with me, so I said goodnight to Karl, gave him a kiss and crawled into bed with Daisy in the guest room, falling fast asleep.

During the night, I woke up with a fright. My mind raced and my heart beat so loud I was sure that it would wake Daisy up! I was drenched in sweat, and it took me a few moments to get myself together.

Where was I? Was Karl ok?

I suddenly realised that I had had the most horrific dream that Karl had died; it was so real that I had tears rolling down my face when I woke! But I was fine and I was safe in bed with my little Daisy.

I checked my phone, it was 4.50 am. *Go back to sleep, Susy, it was just a dream*, I told myself. I lay there for about ten minutes and then decided to check on Karl.

I crept through the house when I heard Karl say, 'Susy, I can't breathe properly and I can't move. I am in so much pain'.

'Oh my God! Are you ok?' I said.

'I don't know. I can only breathe at about 5% lung capacity and I'm really scared. I have also got crippling pains in my chest and stabbing pains when I breathe.'

Instinctively I quickly went over to Karl, helped him up and made him walk around. After a while he said that it was starting to ease as he walked around. I got some painkillers for him and made him a hot water bottle. I gave him some water and then put the fire on for him as he was freezing. He sat by the fire shaking, and I wrapped him in a blanket and put the hot water bottle on his side.

'It's much better. It's still painful but moving around has helped. How come you are up?' Karl asked.

'I just had a dream that you died, and it worried me so much that I had to come down and check that you were ok,' I said.

The painkillers kicked in after about fifteen minutes and made Karl drowsy. He eventually dozed off, convincing me that he was fine and that he probably just had the same virus as the children and me.

It was now 6.00 am, and one by one the children got up. Daisy and Flynn were better and, as usual, Seren was fine. She amazed me that whenever we got ill, she never did! She was so resilient to illness and never seemed to get sick (apart from all the usual behavioural dramas). I dropped Daisy and Seren off at school and then came home with Flynn to check on Karl.

Later that day, Karl had a meeting at home, so I kept Flynn in the playroom with me so they wouldn't be disturbed. I sat on the playroom floor with the rain bouncing off the ceiling, and as Flynn played, it was then that I had an epiphany! I never really understood or new what an epiphany was until that moment. All I knew was that I had an idea and I had to do it.

In that moment, I realised that I wanted to share our experience with other parents, and start a positive ADHD movement! I had no idea how to even start or go about it, but I began typing away in my phone – words, feelings, thoughts … they just kept coming, and I wrote and wrote.

It was Friday, and I loved Fridays! Friday was pizza and movie night with the kids and a glass (or two) of red wine for Mummy.

We sat down to watch the film – pizza in one hand and glass of red in the other. I noticed that Karl was taking strong painkillers again, he was either starting an addiction to those babies or he was in lots of pain.

'Are you ok, Karl, is your leg hurting you at lot?' I asked

'It's not my leg. It's my lung, it's been like this all day, but don't worry, these take the edge off.'

'Karl, that's wrong. I am no doctor but it could be deep vein thrombosis or something much worse, it might have moved up to your lung. I think we should go to the doctors,' I said.

Our doctor's surgery was closed at 1.00 pm on a Friday and it was now 5.45 pm.

'I'll be fine, honestly, don't worry. If it's still bad I will go to the doctors in the morning,' he said.

'No Karl, no way! The dream, the pain in your lung, I am not taking any chances!'

I passed Karl my phone and insisted that he called the other surgery that was about ten minutes drive from us. He spoke with the receptionist who said she had one last appointment, but we had to get there quickly as they were closing in fifteen minutes.

Now sooner than he had gone into the doctor's surgery, Karl came hobbling back out. 'The doctor thinks I might be having a pulmonary embolism. He wants you to drive me to the hospital straightaway. I will be ok, it's just a precaution; I will be fine.'

As we drove, Karl Googled 'pulmonary embolism', and as he read out each one of the symptoms, he had every single one. We said very little on the way to the hospital; we knew it could mean 'death' and we were both petrified but we kept saying to each other: 'You will be fine', 'I will be fine'.

I dropped Karl off at the Emergency Department and headed home with the children. I felt awful leaving him but I didn't think the Emergency

Department on a Friday night with three little ones would be the right answer either.

Seren was starting to panic and was getting agitated, which was understandable. I prayed all the way home, in fact, we all did – Seren and Daisy said a little prayer too. They had no idea what was going on, but it's not every day that you drop your daddy off at the hospital, so they knew something was wrong.

I got home and managed to get them both to bed, promising them that everything would be ok.

Pete's wife, Marie, came over to stay with the children, and I rushed back to the hospital. I sat on the edge of Karl's bed holding his hand when the doctor came over to see us.

In his charming, enigmatic Irish voice he said, 'Well, Karl, you could have died, but hey you didn't!' The doctor then told us that the night before when Karl couldn't breathe, clots had gone through his heart and into his lungs. He explained that if he stayed at home another night, he would have probably died.

It's crazy how it all happened – one minute Karl was healthy and the next minute we could have lost him. I felt like a rabbit in the headlights again, suddenly all the problems with Seren seemed insignificant. Seren's daddy could have died, my soul mate and best friend … gone.

We felt so lucky that we just silently hugged. In the past, this would have been a time where I would have bawled my eyes out, but the bloody Sertraline wouldn't let me. Karl silently shed a few tears on my shoulder, but there I was like the bloody 'Ice Queen', not one single solitary tear. I had absolutely nothing!

Karl stayed in the hospital that night and most of the next day and then he left armed with more painkillers and now some blood thinners to add to the mix.

I have given the pharmaceutical companies a bit of a tough time in this book, but with a twist of fate, they ended up saving us both. Without medication, I would have cried myself into a deep, dark bout of depression. Without medication, Karl would surely have died. So medication does have a place, and I am eternally grateful for this.

Diary entries during this time

22 August

Daddy has a DVT clot in his leg that moved to his lung. I had to take him to the hospital. Seren's behaviour has taken a massive nosedive. She's screaming, slamming doors, threatening to cut all her hair off. She is becoming very anxious, very agitated and defiant – this is hard! ADHD kids cannot cope with change, illness, worry, doubt. If we are to become great parents at managing ADHD, we have to create a safe house as much as possible. She's become so defiant about gluten and dairy – I wonder if there are any videos for kids to watch.

Maybe take out gluten from a young age and then it's the norm? Rough day today, I'm exhausted, stressed and worried. I'm ill with a cough and cold too! Help! :-(

I am so glad Karl is ok though. :-)

3 September

So much to say and not much time. Life is pretty crazy at the moment so I will bullet point:

- The school thinks Seren isn't making friends, and as the class so small, there is little opportunity for her to make any friends.
- The children can't forget what happened at the party and Seren has been 'labelled'.
- Therefore, she is going to find it hard to make friends – 'mud sticks.'
- I have mixed feelings about moving her as she is the happiest she has been since we arrived here eighteen months ago.
- She's happier, calmer and content.
- She's learning.
- I am sick of the long school drive in the mornings!
- Maybe we should look elsewhere?
- Maybe look at schools that specialise in ADHD management?

Seren's birthday

Seren's birthday was on 24th August, but as Daddy had been sick, and life was running at a million miles an hour, we decided to postpone the party for a couple of weeks. Given what happened at the last party, I needed to keep it really small and make sure there was no sugar!

It had been a few months since the last party and Seren was desperate to have some friends over for a small gathering. She helped me make some invitations and then she gave them out the next day. We only asked the four girls from her group, but sadly, only one replied. The mum that had called me the day after the last party sent me a text: 'We will be there, love. We will be there for you'. As I said briefly, she had her own personal journey with ADHD and she understood it, she got it; she knew how it felt as a mother – it was heartbreaking.

One of the other mums did send me a message saying that her daughter could come but she would have to stay at the party. I got it, I really did, but I knew in my heart that not one of the mums wanted their daughters to come. It was horrible. I had always thrown the best parties for Seren. I had always gone to such an effort and made her birthday cakes, also making a theme for each year – even Karl and I would dress up. I never imagined that it would come to this.

Weirdly, a week before the party, Seren came down with the flu. I have never been so happy to have the flu in our family. This was the perfect excuse to the cancel the party. So, we spent Seren's birthday at home – just us. We were all quite sick, so together as a family we shared pizza and a huge chocolate cake. Karl filmed us all singing 'happy birthday' to Seren as I walked into the dining room with the cake. Moments after Seren blew out her candles, Karl asked her, 'So how do you feel on your eighth birthday, Seren?'

'I feel happy. My mummy told me to always believe in myself, I didn't for a while, but now and do and that makes me happy,' she said.

Tears fell silently from my face as I cut the cake and I smiled not only from my face, but also from my heart. We had turned such a corner with little Seren. Gone was the scared, hyperactive, crazy, defiant little girl – here before us sat a miracle. And this miracle was called 'Seren'.

The thing that amazed me about Seren was her resilience; she told me regularly that her friends would have play dates and parties and that she was never invited. She said she wished that they would invite her too, but she was ok with it. Of course, hearing this broke my heart.

Seren was in a small group and they ate morning tea together, had lunch together and played together in the playground. Well, three of them did but they would often leave Seren out. They were sweet girls and, although there was never any real bullying, I feel they struggled to accept her into the group, as Seren was different. However, Seren is Seren! She may always have these social problems, so I guess in some way these situations better prepare her for life, as life can be cruel.

Seren was hyper and impulsive; she would fidget and lose concentration. She would go crazy with excitement at lunchtime, would climb trees and run around until her face was bright red. But, she was also loyal, caring, kind and giving, yet so many of these things were never recognised.

Seren used to make pictures and bracelets and take them to school for her friends and sometimes the teacher. She used to take books and teddies and be continually giving things to other children. I guess she just wanted to feel loved, to feel accepted.

She was such fun too. The boys loved her because she was always full-on, playing basketball, kicking the ball, chasing games, rough play – she was a bit of a tomboy! She would always make lots of friends at the park. She was the crazy one, the zany one who would be doing the scariest things in the park – only Seren could make the local park look like a 'Cirque du Soleil' show!

Asked to leave

At the park, Seren's antics frightened the life out of me, but I also found her mesmerising. There was nothing that she couldn't do. The girl had no fear!

But unfortunately, everyone at school saw was a child who couldn't sit still and was hyperactive. It wasn't the school's fault, and it wasn't the parents', it was my fault for choosing the wrong type of schooling for Seren, but I believe everything happens for a reason. For a child like Daisy, the Montessori education was perfect, but we came to learn that Seren needed a more structured and strict schooling environment.

I believe that Seren's teacher, Diane, helped me to save Seren. She was a beautiful lady who gave me so much support and love at a time when I desperately missed my family and friends. She was very patient and kind to Seren, and was always so positive about her. She told me, 'I predict great things for Seren. She really is one-of-a-kind and will be so interesting to watch'. The teaching assistant was also a great help to Seren too, and I still only have a positive view of Seren's time at the Montessori school.

Many wouldn't see it like that because in the end we were kindly asked to reconsider Seren's schooling. At the time it was crushing, but I am so glad that we left when we did. Seren needed a fresh start and so did I, we all did, and it ended up being one of the best decisions that we ever made. I really feel that the school had Seren's best interests at heart and I am so thankful to the school for the friendly push!

Still learning ...

We have learnt so much as a family over the last eighteen months, but the one thing that I still don't understand is why medication is the first response. I don't understand why medication is being handed out to any child who appears to have ADHD.

I don't agree that these kids should be made to feel that something is wrong with them, that they are naughty and stupid. It is so damaging and causes tremendous anxiety for them, which then causes the ADHD to become worse.

It is still a perception of many experts that you can just give a child a pill and it will make everything better, but that's not always the answer, there is so much more that is needed to be done than just taking medication. I feel that parents should be given more information, more support and more guidance, and that medication should be a last resort.

We are a complex society now, and kids are not allowed to be kids anymore. They don't want to climb trees anymore, play with conkers or make dens, they want to play on computer games, iPads, iPhones, take selfies, and even from such an early age we are teaching them that image is important. We are all to blame.

I once read an article that talked about this in more detail. It mentioned that we needed to address the complex issues that contribute to behavioural, emotional, and learning problems in children. It discussed 'pseudo-ADHD', children who look as if they have ADHD but in fact have an environmentally-induced syndrome caused by too much time spent on electronic connections and not enough time spent on human connections — family dinner, bedtime stories, walks in the park, playing outdoors with friends or relatives, time with pets, buddies, extended family, and other forms of non-electronic connection. Pseudo-ADHD is a real problem; the last thing a child with pseudo-ADHD needs is Ritalin. The article went on to say that above all, children need a loving, safe, and richly-connected childhood and that over time, medication becomes a less important force in a child's improvement and that human connections become even more powerful. It is good and heartening to know that human connection – love – works wonders over time. Love is our most powerful and under-prescribed 'medication'. It's free and infinite in supply, and doctors most definitely ought to prescribe it more.[23]

Children need love

The Pseudo-ADHD argument may stand for many children, but Seren had lots of human connections. We had just moved to Australia, so there was lots of outdoor play, swimming, playing in the park and at the beach. She didn't play computer games and we limited her TV time to about sixty minutes per day, with iPad time at the weekends only.

Diet also plays a huge role. Often children lack vitamins and minerals as our soil now is so depleted, plus you have the ridiculous amounts of chemicals that are in the very things that we nurture our children with – shampoos, body wash, toothpaste, washing powder. The list goes on and on, and don't get me started on the amount of 'can cause behavioural problems in children' additives that are in foods such as crisps and rice cakes.

It is so hard now for parents as we are fighting a war that we don't even know; it's a silent war and the governments are doing very little to protect our children.

I draw on what I have said before – 'ADHD children are hard to love'. Many may argue with me over this, many may agree, but it's certainly how I felt. However, it took me a long time to realise it and to be honest with myself.

That night that Seren told the babysitter, 'Mummy doesn't love me'. It broke my heart. I talked to Seren and she said, 'Mummy, you don't love me; you love Flynn and Daisy but you and Daddy don't love me'.

I had to do something. I had to make a change. I had to make Seren realise that I did love her, more than anything.

I remember my first love and how my heart was utterly shattered when it ended – I think we can all remember our first love ending, and like the song says, 'the first cut is the deepest'; it's so true!

How awful it must have felt for Seren to feel that Karl and I didn't love her, to be a child and to feel so unloved, so sad, so worthless. It makes me so sad to think how she must have felt, and all I did was continually take her to see experts, when all she ever needed was me. She needed Karl and me to love her and hold her, just as we did when she was a beautiful, innocent newborn baby.

At the end of the day, ADHD – Attention-Deficit-Hyperactivity-Disorder – is just a made up name to explain different types of children and adults.

I believe in ADHD, and have learnt through this whole process that if it's channelled in the right way, these kids, these adults, can be awesome! Wouldn't it be great if we could empower these children, love them with abundance, raise their confidence, lift their spirits and make them realise that they are intelligent, amazing, creative and gifted, and that they are on this Earth because they are going to do something great.

Our lives changed forever ...

The day we did this with Seren was the day that our lives changed forever and, more importantly, it was the day that Seren's behaviour started to get better!

Seren and I were in the car; it was winter in Perth and the rain was beating so hard on the windscreen that I could hardly see the road ahead, but the road ahead for Seren was going to change – I knew it, I could feel it, and for the first time I could see it.

We pulled up outside our house and I stopped the car. I faced Seren, held her hands and looked her straight in the eyes. I told her that it was over. I told her that we would not be seeing any more doctors, any more psychologists, and although we didn't know for sure, she probably did have ADHD and that I probably had it too.

I told her all about Richard Branson and Walt Disney and I told her about Einstein and I said, 'You know what Seren, some of the most talented, artistic, creative, amazing people that ever lived had ADHD too, so I reckon that's a great thing'.

I told her how amazing she was, how artistic she was, how brave and resilient she was and how I was so proud to be her mummy. I couldn't finish what I was saying as Seren hugged me so tight and started to cry. She said, 'Mummy, thank you, thank you, so, so much. I love you, Mummy'.

I cried and she cried and then the sun burst through the window of the car and it was a moment that I will never, ever forget. At that moment, what I said to her changed her, it changed our relationship and Seren's future went from dark to light.

Seren was so down on herself; she'd had so many kicks and negativity from Karl and me, from teachers, family, friends, and peers over the years.

She was so confused and didn't know how to act, how to be, how to behave. She was lost and so was I, but after that day, things started to change.

The beauty in her

Once upon a time, all I ever found in Seren's notebooks were messages about how much she hated me, how much she hated Daddy. It made me miserable, thinking that I must have been an awful mum for her to write such things in her notebook.

Weeks after our conversation in the car, Seren's behaviour started to change. Karl and I began to receive the most beautiful notes from her. She would leave them all over the house, and if that didn't speak volumes then I don't know what would. Her behaviour could still be up and down but she was doing so much better – it was a miracle.

> To Mummy I love you
> To Mummy you are the best in the hole wide welded. You are the bestest Mummy every wot has bine. I love it wen we spend time together. And I think you deserve some think amazing. You are the love of my life, you sparkle like a star. You lite up the welde.

Diary entries during this time

7 September
We have a changed little girl! Unbelievable! Looking now at a community school, it seems like a Montessori school but with more art and outdoor nature play, which Seren loves. We think it might be perfect for Seren. Seren is doing well with the essential oils and I love them too! I would love to try and help other mamas going through this – maybe do some free eBooks. Lots to plan!

14 September
One week later and OMG we have a different child! Wild, anxious, clawed hands and feet, screaming, spitting, scared and being a night- mare at school, grabbing at Daisy and Flynn, the list is endless!

She is refusing to have an iron test but I am worried that maybe she lacks iron again. It is all starting again, I am so afraid of this, and I am so tired of it all too!

She has sworn in school and is being an absolute nightmare.

I am planning on sending her to our local school but I am so unsure how this will go. I have tried so hard, but this is so difficult. I think it's us talking about the change at school, I believe that it's causing her significant anxiety. Just use essential oils tomorrow? Maybe try different ones!

Letting things go

Even though we were looking at alternative private schools, we were also considering sending Seren to our local, public primary school. Pete and Marie's girls go there and they only have great things to say about it. Marie said it was quite strict, but I liked that. The more I read about ADHD, the more I realised that Seren may thrive with this type of schooling.

Their eldest daughter, who was seven, was a beautiful little soul. She was so sweet and played well with Seren. Pete and Marie have been great with Seren. At times, they found it hard as our new way of parenting was now to, 'let things go', 'don't sweat the small stuff', 'ignore the bad, praise the good'.

I also found this way of parenting a lot harder for me than for Karl; remember I was brought up with a 'mighty one', so saying nothing to Seren when she was rude and obnoxious was difficult.

I once read an article from a parenting expert who wrote that even if your teenager is swearing as they tidy their room, at least they are doing it. They cannot help their mood, as their hormones are raging and they are trying to figure it out, but at least they are tidying their room, which means progress! I try and think of this at all times and think of Seren as a teenager, thankfully we don't have the swearing yet, but it will come, that I know.

Pete and Marie explained to their daughter all about Seren's personality. They told her that when Seren ran off and wanted to be on her own, that she was not to follow her but just wait for her to come back. They explained that when Seren got crazy and hyper, she was to just go with it and let her be; that when she said silly things or acted impulsively, not to worry and just be her friend.

Over the months, I have watched their relationship grow and I now see that there is a real friendship there. She has such an appreciation and under- standing of Seren's personality and one day, when Seren is older, she will come to realise what a wonderful friend she is.

The lemonade stall

One particular day, Seren had been with Jade for the day when she came home with the biggest lemons that I had ever seen, from Jade's garden.

It was a cold, grey, winter day in Perth, but Seren said she wanted to make a lemonade stall. She made the sign and then we set about to make 'sugar free' (of course) lemonade! We took the lemonade, the sign, the table, the cups and straws outside onto the drive, and we all stood there in the cold! I think people felt sorry for us, as Karl sat with his 'peg leg' in a cast and his crutches next to him. It was a real family affair, even Chip joined us!

A few people stopped and then a lovely lady in a car pulled up and bought some lemonade, her name was Della. She was the acting deputy head of the local public school that we were thinking of sending Seren to.

I have always been one to wear my heart on my sleeve, so we began talking and I started to tell her about the Montessori school, about Seren and my confusion as were to send Seren. Della said, 'Come and see me in the morning and we will talk about it. You can move her to us straightaway at the start of the new term, if you like.'

Just like that, God sent an angel! I will never forget that day, we were so happy. I was researching all different types of schools, going to open days, school tours, and all the time the perfect school was sitting just metres away from us (how lucky we were that the school was only a five-minute walk away)!

Keeping it mainstream

One thing that I have learnt about ADHD is that often the best type of schooling is mainstream. I have heard that some private schools will often portray offering the best kind of support for ADHD children, but very soon you will have the other 'paying customers' complaining about the ADHD child and you may find yourselves being asked to leave. If you can find a good public school who can offer you support for your child with IEP

(Independent Education Plan) additional assistance, and (if need be) the support of a school psychologist, then you have a winner!

Karl and I went the very next morning to visit Della. We talked about Seren, our fears, how she was behind in reading and writing, and also the concerns we had about her making friends. With only one week left of this term, we decided that both Seren and Daisy would start the new school after the school holidays.

Seren had been doing better at the Montessori school and we were so proud of her achievements, but she was still struggling to make friends. Unfortunately her small group of friends couldn't forget what had happened at the party and she wasn't getting invited to any other parties or playdates. She was aware of this and it was making her sad. 'Why aren't I invited to anyone's house for a play date or a party, Mummy?' It would break my heart.

The school felt that as Seren was in such a good place, it was a good time to move her. She was calmer and happier and hopefully the transition would be a smooth one.

I found the last day of school emotional, it had so been such a journey with so many ups and downs. Since the party, I had always felt embarrassed and there had been more complaints about Seren's impulsivity from some of the other mums. I felt sad to be leaving some wonderful friends that I had made at the school, but I was so glad for Seren that she could start afresh. We could wipe the slate clean and start again.

Diane and the teaching assistant told me how fond they were of Seren. They said they found her fascinating and that she would do something great in life. I watched them as they hugged her on the last day and told her how proud they were of her. Diane had been a great support to us all, and I will be forever grateful for her love, care and support.

Shortly after leaving the Montessori school, Seren gave me this letter.

To Mummy,
From this day I promise I will be an amazing help to you. This is how I can make up for all the bad things I have done. I know that I can do it, I promise. Let's forget about all the bad times that we had together and think about all the good times and let's start with that, shall we?
Lots of love Seren xxx

A real holiday!

A week later we went camping down to Margaret River with Pete, Marie and their girls. We had had some pretty horrific holidays over the last eighteen months with Seren, but she was in her element here at the caravan park. It was only a small caravan and camping park, and she loved it so much because she had freedom. She could swim, climb trees, run around and scoot to her heart's content. When Seren was happy, the whole family was happy.

We had some initial issues with Seren – she would run away for the first couple of hours after we arrived. We also lost her at one point and were all running around the holiday camp, and once again I found myself running up and down on the beach screaming, 'Seren, Seren, Seren', but we found her again, as we always did … up a tree!

She was a bit defiant, a bit cheeky, a bit hyper, but we dealt with it; it was nothing compared to what we had been through.

Another light bulb moment (God, how many is that now?)

It was during this holiday that I had my most significant 'light bulb' moment. We had changed lots of things to help Seren with her ADHD, but one of the biggest things I believe we had to ensure was that we showed her that we loved her unconditionally. We also had to realise that she wasn't being difficult to upset us. It was nothing personal. It was just the way she was made.

I thought of my past and my toxic relationship with my own mother.

I thought of my relationship with my dad, and although I am now very close to him, he almost washed his hands of me when I was younger, as he was so fed up with my behaviour.

I remembered how at fifteen I had left home. I had fallen in with the wrong crowd, left school with not one single exam to my name and was spiralling out of control. My mother had disowned me; my father had had enough, and then I remembered who had saved me – it was my stepmum, Karen.

She had only met me about a year before, but she had been so kind to me. However, it took me twenty years to recognise this. What is it they say – better late than never (and I have always been late for everything)!

I left the kids and Karl playing on the beach and then ran back to the caravan to send Karen a message. I was crying as I wrote it and could hardly see the keyboard as I typed.

Thank you so much for the love and nurturing that you showed me when you first met me. It makes my cry thinking about what you did, as I must have been so hard to love. You are a beautiful soul and, if I am honest, you saved me. I know we are two very different spirits and I drive you mad at times (as you do me, hehe) but I want you to know that you have a very special place in my heart. I love you dearly, you are not my blood mother, but you have been the only true mum that I have ever had.

Thank you so much for everything you have done, I appreciate it so much. Thank you so much for the support you have given me with Seren. I am a better mum because of you. Please know that you are my family, you always have been and always will be a huge part of our life. I am eternally grateful for your love! Love you millions. xxxxx

And her reply:
Thank you for that. Know that I truly love you and I am very proud of you, my daughter. xxxxx

If Karen hadn't shown me love, compassion, and given me a secure home, a safe place, I don't know where I would be today.

I had always felt that I saved myself, but now I see that I was never alone. I had someone holding my hand, someone loving me, someone guiding me the whole time.

Karen and I have had our ups and downs over the years – we are very different, chalk and cheese, but I can never forgot what she did for me. Many would have given up on me and walked away. She didn't, and I was so glad that I didn't give up on Seren.

Life with Seren will always be a rollercoaster ride, but to medicate her, dampen down her spirit, her determination, her zest for life, no-one has the right to do that.

You have to change your thinking

Seren moved schools and the transition went really well. I honestly wouldn't have believed it, if someone had told me. She loved the walk to school. She loved the school, the teachers, and I couldn't believe the transformation in her, it was a miracle.

I prayed so hard that everything would be ok for Seren in the new school. I never thought myself to be particularly religious but Karen's family is Catholic and very religious, the priest even goes for Sunday lunch to Grandma's house. Karen would tell me how every Sunday, Grandma, Auntie Vera and Father Martin would all pray for Seren. I remember speaking to my grandma on the phone and thanking her for praying for Seren, 'Please thank Father Martin and tell him a miracle has happened, Grandma'. She was so happy and still prays for Seren every Sunday at Church.

One thing that I have learnt is if you want to change your future, you have to change your thinking. I was so fearful that Seren was seriously mentally ill. I worried that she may have something really wrong with her, like bipolar or schizophrenia. But little did I realise that the more I manifested these feelings, the more I was drawing it to me, I was making these thoughts inside my head as big as monsters.

Seren was so lucky that her new teacher was a fantastic, recently-graduated teacher. I had a meeting with her two weeks after Seren started school and she told me that Seren was very bright. She explained that when she taught the lesson, Seren would continually draw pictures. However, if she asked her to repeat what she had said, Seren could tell her word for word, even though she had been drawing the whole time.

I loved her for this, and I remembered what Pete had said to me once. When he was a child, he found that he could only concentrate if he looked out the window, yet the teacher would get angry at him for daydreaming. Again I go back to the sentiment that we have to change how we teach these children.

Seren aged eight

Seren is just eight, and although I feel like we have learnt so much, I somehow feel that we are just at the beginning of this journey.

They say it takes a village to raise a child, and this is so true.

I hope that by sharing our story, I can help to create that village – that community – that all ADHD parents need.

Chapter Eleven

Learning to live, love and laugh
with ADHD

Once upon a time, it felt like we were just existing, we had no answers, no solutions and no hope. Then a miracle happened, a wish was granted, a prayer was heard, and finally our beautiful little butterfly left her cacoon. Only then could we see how truly beautiful she was.

Correspondence and diary entries during this time

5 November

Hi Susy,

I have been meaning to drop you an email long before this to see how Seren is going.
We have had three new little boys begin and two more little girls transitioning today so life has been busy in class.
The children are at the library now so I promised myself to write a quick hello.
We really hope she is loving being close to home etc.
Lots of thoughts, Diane xx

19 November

Hi Diane,

I am so sorry this is late; I must have replied to you about twenty times in my head! Seren is doing great and I honestly can't believe the transformation, it's like a miracle has happened!

Firstly, it's not just the school, you were amazing Diane, and I will be so grateful to you forever. You helped me realise at such an early age who Seren is, and how she functions, and I believe that this would never have happened in a mainstream school.

I am so glad that we are equipped with this knowledge before she enters her teens, and I just want to thank you so much for all your time, support and love that you gave Seren and the rest of the family.

Seren is really lucky to have a great teacher that understands her like you did, it made the transition so much easier. She loves the new class format as well as the art classes and lots of sport! Seren has just done two weeks of swimming and loved it. She also goes to an after-school art class that is on for 1.5 hours, and we still have to prise her away at the end! She is even starting piano lessons, which I never thought she could do.

I am writing a book about the whole journey and I'm really hoping that it can help other parents who are going through a similar thing with their child because there are lots of them. I am so happy that we have managed to do it without medication as well, as that never really sat well with me, as you know.

Seren is making friends too, which is so great. She has just had her little friend over for a play, and they were like two peas in a pod. One of my good friend's daughters goes to the school, so there has been lots of love and support for Seren. I feel so grateful!

Hope all is great with you guys.

Love, Susy xx

22 November

We went to friends for lunch and Seren watched TV by herself. Before we left, Seren stole the bubbles off Lyla and refused to give it back. It was also so hard to get her into the car; however, we could feel it happening and managed to stay calm, keeping it together, and left before all hell broke loose.

We got home and Seren wanted to sleep in my bed. Overall the day went really well, so we only praised her on her good behaviour. We did refer to the 'bubble incident' but mainly we focused on the positives.

23 November

Seren woke this morning and was really tired. We had a busy weekend and I did feel that it would hit her today! I got the 'Zen' music on, and she ate breakfast. We were all walking on eggshells because it could kick off at any second. She got dressed and then went off to do her mindful- ness art, which is great to keep her focused in the mornings. For me, I don't allow the kids to watch TV before school, I find it gets the brain firing in all sorts of directions. I am lucky though as Karl is around before school, so I realise that mums have got to do whatever they can! And when Karl isn't home, or I am pre-menstrual or having a really bad day, then I reach for the remote, but I try my best not to.

Just as Seren was about to leave for school, I saw that she was frustrated. Karl shouted at her to grab her bag, and she walked out of the house ignoring him, grabbing her scooter and started to scoot off up the road. I saw him getting angry. I calmly told Seren that I was taking her money out of the jar, but she could earn it straight back if she was good for Dad on the way to school.

We stayed calm; she stops scooting. I told Karl to leave it, using the hand signal across the neck – this is something that we both use A LOT to support each other when we see the other one is losing it!

Note to self – don't sweat the small stuff, focus on the positive, remain calm.

24 November

Seren woke up in a bad mood, and as usual I tried to figure it out. Is it because she has been asked to take a toy to school today, or is it because she has to take money to the school for the fair, most kids would be so excited but to Seren she is in utter turmoil!

I sent her to her room, screaming, hitting, kicking, but she went. No time-out anymore, just 'calm down time'. She has to understand that she can't act like that in the family unit, and if she does she will be excluded and will need time away from us all to calm down.

Seren moans every time I give her food at mealtimes. She hates the way it looks, the texture, the bowl is wrong, the spoon is wrong – I tell myself to just ignore it or I will have a never-ending battle. Smile through it Susy, rise above it!

Off my antidepressants

I decided to come off the antidepressants on 13th October (my lucky number), and two days after my thirty-ninth birthday. I had been taking a very low dose for almost five months – they had served their purpose, they had helped me through some dark times, but now it was time to say goodbye!

Am I embarrassed that I took antidepressants to cope with my daughter's behaviour? Yes, which is why only a few people know about it, although I am learning to come to terms with it.

Do I regret it? Hell no! And you want to know why I don't regret it ... because I realised what it was like to take medication. I felt the benefits and also the side effects and then I gradually took myself off it after five months.

Why did I do this when I was advised to stay on it for 6–12 months? Because I realised that, I was slowly starting to become addicted. Not addicted in a physiological way, but in an emotional way.

When travelling back to the UK, I met up with my good friends for lunch. I had told my best friend that I was on antidepressants, but I hadn't told the other girls. As we were driving to the restaurant, I suddenly remembered that I had forgotten to take my morning pill! I almost wanted to ask my best friend to stop the car and turn back, but I couldn't as I was too embarrassed. So you know what I did? When we got the restaurant, I ordered a large glass of wine to take the edge off my anxiety!

After this, I made sure that I had my tablets in my bag, at home and in the car, just in case I forgot to take it. I had only been on these antidepressants for a couple of months, but here I was starting an addiction. It was an addiction because I felt that I couldn't cope or function without them. I had lost the belief in myself that I was able to do this on my own, and for me that is the start of addiction right there!

However, at the time, I was glad of the support that I had from the medication, but I am also now so happy to be off it.

I now dose myself in essential oils every day, take supplements, exercise and meditate. All the things I do with Seren, I do with myself.

Why? Because she is a mini version of me, and like the old saying goes, 'The apple doesn't fall very far from the tree'.

It's been a long road for both of us, but I am finally learning that my racing thoughts, full-on personality and the ability to never, ever stop are all just part of who I am. It's my personality and I wouldn't have it any other way. I have finally learnt to accept myself, to take the time to meditate, relax, eat really well, drink less coffee, accept anxiety, and to love myself, warts and all (most of the time anyway).

Understanding my personality has been key to helping Seren realise who she is. And it has allowed me to help her stand tall and be proud of the beautiful human being that she is, and I am so lucky to be her mama.

My ADHD

I have mentioned before that one of the main things for me on a personal level was to realise that I probably have ADHD myself. Looking further into my family tree, I am pretty convinced that my dad has ADHD too (sorry Dad).

It made me realise so much about myself and why I acted the way I did when I was younger. Memories came flooding back of school reports that said, 'Susy is very bright and has the ability, but lacks concentration'. I remember every report from every teacher had the same message – I lacked concentration!

I thought about how I have always been described as hyper, excitable, a bottle of pop, a butterfly fluttering everywhere. And when I was younger, friends would often say I was weird because I oddly blurted things out without thinking, often getting myself into trouble.

I thought how, when I tidy the house, I tidy it like a crazy person running from room to room tidying and cleaning simultaneously. I am not able to finish one room as I am thinking about what's needed to be done in the next room. I tell you what, though, I get it all done and probably in record time compared to most people.

I cook quickly, eat quickly, drink quickly, and talk quickly; in fact, I do everything quickly and I am unable to do it any other way. I used to feel very different to other people, and I would cry to my husband (who was then my boyfriend at age twenty-five) that I was different to other people. I would see friends and peers almost floating through life with minimal problems. I had debt, would crash cars, fall out with friends, and would drink way too much (I was a bit reckless, to say the least).

Positively positive!

Let's talk about some positives! I was super happy, friendly to everyone, inquisitive, kind, caring and full of ideas! There was nothing that I couldn't do, no career that I couldn't achieve, and no place too far to travel!

I have moved numerous times; I think the last count was nineteen homes since I was born. I've moved all over the UK, once living in London for 12 months before hating it and moving back home. I have travelled everywhere, even moving to Australia. But despite all the positives, with this type of personality came stress, anxiety and lots of emotions.

Today I am a million times better and I have learnt how to manage myself, and my feelings (well almost).

I am finally settled and happy with life – six months ago I couldn't have said that. I was depressed, anxious and petrified. It was such a scary time, but I realise that it taught me something – it taught me how to be a better wife, a better daughter, a better mother.

My whole life suddenly made sense and for the first time, 'I got it'! I got me.

The rest of my family

Karl is the complete opposite of me; he is relaxed, chilled, super happy and positive. Our four-year-old Daisy is completely like her daddy. She is pragmatic, wise, kind and gentle, and everyone who meets her falls in love with her.

Her younger brother, two-year-old Flynn, is Daisy's best friend. They have the occasional fight, but mainly they spend endless days playing together. They share a room (even though Daisy has her own room, she refuses to sleep in it) and they are true buddies. Flynn is Daisy's shadow, and she is his teacher. I watch her, mesmerised, constantly teaching him how to do things – look for ants or bugs, go down the slide or jump over the waves when we are at the beach. The reason that I find them fascinating is that Seren has never been like that. She likes to control everything. She doesn't allow others to participate in games (it's her way or the highway), she isn't very good at playing with her siblings, gets very angry, has outbursts and absolutely doesn't have any empathy.

Although, I have to say that recently she has started being kind to her sister, teaching her to swim, guiding her, loving her, and it's beautiful to watch. To some families that may be normal, to us it's a miracle.

Our life with Seren will always have bumps in the road, but she is learning to manage her ADHD – the good, the bad, and the ugly – one step at a time! We are all finally learning to live, love and laugh with ADHD.

Diary entry during this time

2 December

Seren's behaviour is starting to get bad again. Defiant, running away, scared, crying, tantrums, screaming ...

I have been shouting a bit more than usual, and I am noticing that it is having an adverse effect on the children. I must stop it!

Seren today ran off and hid at the bus stop before school; it was really hard, and I felt stressed and at the end of my tether.

Afterwards, Karl took her to school. He couldn't get her out of the car, so instead of fighting with her, he parked and got out of the car and sat down next to a tree outside the school. He said he had to sit there for about two minutes before Seren finally got out of the car. She stated that she was sorry, that she loved him, and then she skipped off into school. We had a stressful morning with Seren. It was not a good time of the month for me, and I should have cancelled the park date with my friend that morning.

I could feel that I was stressed, and I have learnt that the children pick up on this. We went to the park and Flynn hit a little girl, then Daisy pushed Flynn off the wall. I told her off and then she started screaming that she wanted an ice-cream. I said no so she started hitting me – my cup was so full (metaphorically speaking) that I just didn't have the patience this morning for this!

Daisy is usually so good, but as Seren's behaviour worsens, so does Daisy's – there we go again with the learnt behaviour!

When I look back on this diary, I didn't write in it throughout October. This shows me how good Seren's behaviour was during that month.

For example, when Seren was on Risperidone I didn't make one note in this book!

I always start writing when Seren's behaviour is bad! Karl is convinced it's due to the iron, and she lacks iron again, so here's the plan ...

Plan
- Thursday – Seren blood test to confirm if she is low in iron
- Naturopath – get her to check the supplements that I am giving Seren
- No TV in the morning – there is a definite link with bad behaviour
- Love-bombing!
- I am going to spend some time this weekend with the kids separately and love-bomb them like crazy!

She is just different, and that's ok

I have absolutely loved writing this book – it's been hugely cathartic.

In some chapters I have laughed at the craziness of it all, and other times, my heart has almost burst with pride when I reflect on how far Seren has come.

At times it's been so hard to write, and I have found myself in constant floods of tears. I found that I was reliving it all over again, and I found that really difficult. But overall, it's lifted a lot of baggage that I was carrying around on a daily basis.

Sometimes, I feel that we are at the end of a very dark tunnel, and I never want to go back through it again. I only want to carry on travelling along the little bumpy roads – those little bumps I can handle!

But life isn't like that, and I have no idea what lies ahead for us – for Seren or even Daisy and Flynn, for that matter. But what I have realised is that it is my absolute duty as a parent to empower, love and build my children's self-esteem until no-one can ever knock them down.

Seren has already had so many knocks in her short eight years of life. She has been made to feel like a freak, feel naughty, feel weird, feel unloved, feel unliked, feel that she isn't smart, and the worst – she has been made to feel different.

Yes, she is different, she is different because she sees the world in a different light and because of this, most people will think she is different. However, she is outgoing, curious, fun, intelligent, creative, focused, and has boundless energy that could even make a greyhound jealous. And because of this, she needs loving, she needs empowering, she needs building up.

I now finally understand, appreciate and respect that Seren isn't great with change, and there is so much changing in her life right now, which is sending her into a spin!

If I had carried on with the medication plan for Seren, she would now be medicated on Ritalin and Risperidone or, even worse, Seroquel – a drug that is not approved for children under the age of fourteen (just to clarify, Seren was only seven when she was prescribed it).

Only yesterday, Seren cried so much after school, she was writhing around on the floor screaming. If it had been one year ago, I would have gone straight back to the pediatrician's office. But I didn't, I just said, 'Let it all out Seren, just let it go'.

It took about 3–4 minutes and then she bellowed to me that she needed a hug! I went and sat with her and she lay her head on my knee as I stroked her head. She sobbed, and we talked about what was going on in school. She told me how she was so worried about going into Year Three, she was behind and not like the other children, and she didn't feel ready to move up.

I talked to her about all the positives, how creative she is, how amazing she is at art, at swimming, at dancing, at gymnastics and how much we all loved her. I told her that mummy didn't know what she was doing either and that often I was just flying by the seat of my pants! I told her that as long as she did her best that was all she could do.

She had been trying to do her whole weeks homework on a Monday night, and after realising that she was too tired and couldn't do it, she fell into a heap. Seren can hyper-focus, and the great thing for her (and us) is that she loves words and times tables, so she actually doesn't mind her homework.

Was she a crazed, wild ADHD, ODD kid who needed medicating? Or was she just a little girl who was behind in her reading and writing and who was starting to get nervous because her world was about to change?

She was about to have a new teacher, a new class, new friends and it was all too much for her to cope with. I am finally learning to remember all this about her, as well as learning to recognise how Seren is so sensitive to change.

I strongly believe that if we can get the message out to parents that their children aren't flawed, that they don't always need a label and medication, I believe that we can save generations of children from becoming depressed, medicated, and feeling completely worthless.

Diary entries during this time

10 December

Seren was amazing in the school Christmas concert! We told her that she will know who her teacher will be in Year Three before she finishes school for the summer holidays, she is so happy!

We went away for the weekend to support a friend who was doing the iron man in Busselton. Screaming, hitting, running off, defiant – here we go again, hello old friend!

The change happens when Seren isn't in control, so then how can it be acceptable to put these children on time-out or to punish them.

It's a big thing for ADHD children to be in control, so they know what's happening.

Maybe this is why they control games, play, and their friends. Why should medication change them? It's who they are, which is why so many entrepreneurs and leaders have ADHD.

When I saw a CBT specialist many years ago, she said the one word that I kept saying was 'control'. She noticed straightaway that I was someone who, like Seren, needed to be in control. I am thirty-nine and still the same, so how can I expect a seven-year-old with my genes and ADHD to be any different?

My family are coming over in a matter of days and although I am excited, I am panicking about the change, the unknown, Seren, etc.

23 December

Seren's behaviour has started to worsen again. She has been freaking out, saying the essential oils are burning her skin (they are not), she says they feel weird, and she screams, cries, fights with everyone.

Her defiance is really bad. I am going to make sure she has lots of rest and we will continue to talk about the changes. Could the excitement of Christmas be too much? She is refusing to let me put the oils on her, so I will diffuse them in her room instead. I am going to give her some iron too today, just in case it's that? Her anxiety levels are high, she has had gluten and dairy too, so I will stop that and see how we go.

I have put her in my bed to calm down. The oils aren't stinging, she tells me – she is just freaking out. TV off! The less stimulus, the better. Stay calm, Susy – love her, go outside and scream if need be, throw a tennis ball at the bloody wall, but stay calm! Oils, oils, oils, for me too! My reaction is critical now in these moments! I will go and hug her and tell her that I love her and I am here for her, always. :-)

Being creative

Seren eventually calmed down that day, and then went outside to finish painting her clay mouldings, which she had made a couple of days before. As she painted, I realised that she could happily answer my questions.

Ever since her teacher told me how Seren draws in class when she is talking, I have understood that Seren can communicate better with me when she is creative. Later that day, we talked about our emotions and the film Inside Out. We talked about how she felt about Christmas. She said she was excited, scared and worried. She was worried that Santa wouldn't like her as she has ADHD, she hits her sister, and she is naughty. She also told me that she was worried bout Grandma and Grandad coming to stay, as the last time they came she was really bad.

I focused on the positives and told her how much she was loved, how proud we were of her, how Grandma and Grandad were proud of her too, of everything she had achieved and that Santa would see that too – she had nothing to worry about.

She smiled and said, 'Thank you, Mummy. I love you'.

Note to myself

Always remember that:

- ADHD needs love, not always medication
- Talk, don't shout
- Love, not smack
- All you need is love ...

My perfect note

That afternoon, Seren handed me this note (her spelling isn't the best, but the intention is beautiful).

My Speech

To Mummy I love you
You are the bests friend in the hole wide weld You are the best
You are my hero
You are the love of my life
You are best in the weld
Well done fur all your hord work with your book.

Diary entries during this time

25 December
Christmas Day.
Santa has been and there is so much excitement in the house! Seren opened her presents and she was so happy. I went into Daisy and Flynn's room and they both excitedly opened their presents. Seren then came into the bedroom, sad and disappointed. She didn't receive the clapping dog from Santa, so said, 'Santa hates me. I knew it! He hates me'.
That bloody clapping dog, surely a barking dog is the same, right? Apparently not when you are eight! Seren cried and then was mean to Daisy and Flynn. She made the household quite sombre and stressful! She did come back around and was ok again, but the day was full of highs and lows. She did play with Daisy for a couple of hours and that was beautiful and made me very happy!

30 December
Grandma and Grandad arrived and the children were so excited! Seren's behaviour has been difficult over the past few days; we are finding it hard, but we keep reminding ourselves it's the change!

31 December

Seren's behaviour again is erratic. We are going to a New Year's Eve Party and Seren started to get defiant. 'I'm not going. There will be people there that I don't know. I don't want to go and you can't make me.'

I noticed that today she was very anxious, so I hugged her and told her that sometimes I feel the same when something is new or different and that is completely normal. I told her we should always try new things and try to be excited and positive. I told Seren to come and hug me whenever she felt funny at the party.

Over the night she came up and hugged me about three or four times, each time saying nothing – just a hug and then off she ran. I told her each time that I loved her so much and that I was so proud of her, she then ran off again to play with her friends.

She was fearless

My parents stayed with us for three weeks, and on one of those days we went on a four-hour canoe trip along the river. Seren was amazing, even helping with the paddling and assisting Daisy to do it.

We canoed towards some huge boulders in the river and everyone climbed out of the canoe and clambered onto the rocks. My dad laughed that it was so steep we felt like mountain goats. The guide dived into the water first, followed by Karl, followed by Seren, and all the other people on the trip clapped and cheered.

Seren has no fear! That day, she was totally fearless and jumped in from quite a height without hesitating. I don't think I would have done that at age eight. I don't think I would even do it now (I did jump in that day though).

She swam out of the river, climbed back up the rocks and did it again, in fact she did it several times, her enthusiasm was infectious. And she was in her clothes too, as she had left her bathers in the canoe.

A few days later, Seren did some rock wall climbing and again she was fantastic. Wearing a little harness and no shoes, she climbed the wall to the very top (which Karl told me was impossible to do without the shoes)! She then had a go at doing somersaults on a trampoline, and she didn't just do one somersault, she did several – my amazing, fearless ADHD daughter!

Another time Seren was fearless was when she saved Pete and Marie's daughter, Lily, from drowning.

It was a beautiful hot day and the family had come over for the day to hang out and meet my parents. All the kids were playing in the pool and the adults were standing by the pool, chatting, drinking and watching the kids. We had the music on loud and some inflatables were bobbing around so we couldn't see that the filter was sucking Lily's hair and pulling her down into the water.

Seren saw what happened and straightaway she pulled Lily up out of the water. Her hair was being sucked into the pump so hard that Seren didn't have the strength to pull her out of the water completely, but she did have the strength to keep Lily's head above water and stop her from drowning. She didn't let go and held on as tight as she could, while calmly but firmly shouting, 'Dad, Dad, Lily needs you'.

No-one could hear Seren yelling as the music was so loud and we couldn't see what was happening as the inflatables were in the way. But Seren never let go of Lily, and although it probably all happened very quickly, to Seren it must have seemed like a lifetime!

Lily, as you can imagine, was hysterical. Finally we all noticed what was going on and helped Lily and Seren out of the pool. Everyone was completely devastated and frightened at what could have happened. However, throughout the whole ordeal, Seren never left Lily.

Afterwards, she stayed by Lily's side for quite a while, and I put a movie on for them. Later, Seren came to me to get the essential oils, saying, 'Mummy, I need lavender and coconut oil please'.

I gave Seren the oils and then she gave Lily a lavender foot massage, some water and crisps and looked after her like a little mummy.

For most of Seren's short life, she had been the naughty one, the crazy one, the hyperactive one, the impulsive one, but here she was the calm one, the helpful one, the Hero!

I hope she remembers that day for the rest of her life – I will make sure that she does, because it was the day that Seren saved someone.

Seren didn't need 'saving'

I had spent eighteen months trying to save Seren and then she did the unthinkable! The crazy, hyperactive, defiant, out of control little ADHD girl saved someone's life! And I believe it was because of her determination, her hyper-focus and her quick-thinking, amazing, different little brain that made her do it.

I know that one day Seren will grow up to become something amazing – she has the determination, willpower, resilience and intelligence to go really far. She may not be the best reader or the best speller, but when she finds her passion, there will be no stopping her! I read something once which said ' strong-willed children become adults who change the world, as long as we can hang on for the ride and resist the temptation to 'tame' the spirit out of them. And as hard as it is, I am hanging on for dear life.

When I look back on what happened to Seren, I realise that she was suffering from extreme anxiety, not her ADHD, and didn't need medicating for it. ADHD is a part of who she is. If she were parented, taught and directed in the right way, her ADHD would be her success, not her downfall.

I believe that it's her defiance and her anxiety that will cause the problems, and if we can manage these as a family, by helping and supporting her, I feel that she will have a great life.

Seren needed to be loved – she needed so much love that she could float out of her anxiety. She needed to feel safe, secure and valued. During those tough years, she didn't feel these at all, so she went further and further into an anxiety-filled state, which in children often manifests itself as hyperactivity.

Children are not adults, they are CHILDREN, they believe in the Tooth Fairy, they believe in Father Christmas and they believe in their parents. They need their parents to love, not punish, guide, not control, lift their spirits so high they could take on anything.

I realised that if I wanted to change my child's behaviour, I had to change my own. It has been the hardest thing that I have even done in my life, but I now have the best relationship with my daughter. I have changed the cycle in my family and it's the best thing that I have ever done.

One of the turning points in our relationship was realising that Seren was mirroring me. She is very much like me – she is outgoing, excitable, forgetful, short-tempered, and is so in tune with my mood ... great! That's all I need when I'm having an 'off-day', have less patience, and can fly off the handle at the slightest thing!

We travelled this journey together – had blood tests together, changed our diet together, used essential oils together, and this created a bond between us. I remember I used to feel upset that I gave Seren so much more attention than the other two children. I would have preferred to spend all my time with them, as they were cute, funny and as good as gold. Yet, I spent it with Seren and it drove me crazy as she was insane at times and she was hard to be around.

I am so glad that I invested all that time, as it's paid off ten fold. She is now the funny one, the cute one ... but ... good as gold – I'm not sure she will ever be that (sorry Seren)!

What happens when the kids say no?

I once read about a mother who gave her daughter Ritalin as soon as she woke up. When her daughter then came home from school, she would feed her and then give her sleeping tablets to send her to sleep. This was her life, her existence, and the mother couldn't cope with her daughter's behaviour unless she did this. This mum is not alone, and this is happening to many children right now all over the world.

I am not judging the mother; I know how hard it is, believe me I do. But there will be a day when that child gets old enough to say 'no'. *Then what? What happens then? These kids who we can control with words, with medication, with time-out, with fear, what happens when they become teenagers? What then? What happens when they don't come home, when they turn to drink, drugs, the opposite sex, then what happens?*

I didn't have a relationship with my birth mother, and I hated living at home. My dad had moved out and my home life became a living hell, so at fifteen I packed my bags and walked out, leaving my mother alone. I left school and moved into a bedsit with a group of unemployed, wild, party animals. My life could have spiralled out of control, but it didn't, and I was going to make damn sure that it wouldn't spiral out of control now either.

I think the one thing that made me like a dog with a bone throughout all of this was the constant reminder that I didn't have a relationship with my mother, and how I had struggled with that for most of my life.

This was not going to happen with Seren; I would do anything and everything to make sure that history wasn't going to repeat itself.

Finding their inner genius

I have also learnt that Seren's saviour is art, so I encourage her to do art whenever she can. She goes to an after-school art class and also does various art classes in the school holidays.

She is also fantastic at gymnastics and is an amazing swimmer. She swims with such grace and poise, which always fascinates me as she spends most of the time out of the water being animated and hyperactive.

Many ADHD children are sporty, musical or arty, and if we can help them to realise their potential, this, in turn, will help us, as they will have increased confidence. They also hyper-focus when they enjoy something, but I feel it's important that the focus doesn't just become TV or video games (Seren could quite easily watch TV for an entire day if I let her).

We need to help them find their inner creative genius, as I believe they all have one. They also have great resilience. Can you imagine being told all your life that you are naughty, different, behind in school ... yet these children still try so hard to please everyone because they want to do well.

They also think outside the box and look at the world in a different way, which can be challenging as a teacher when you need your students to be doing the same thing at the same time.

It's important to say here, that in my experience I have found that ADHD children need to have structure and routine and if they don't, this can cause their behaviour to worsen as they become hyperactive and defiant.

A special expert

I have read countless books on ADHD. I have watched numerous experts talk about how the brain works, the lack of dopamine, the difference in the way transmitters speak to each other and how ADHD has comorbid symptoms such as ODD, tics and dyslexia, etc.

There are so many experts with their theories, diets, pills, ideas, concepts and medication.

I haven't got a degree in psychology or psychiatry. I'm not a pediatrician or naturopath, but what I do have is experience, so I hope that my experiences can help other parents and children.

When it comes to dealing with Seren, our beautiful little daughter who is so complex, deep, and often very hard to understand, I consider myself an expert.

It's not unique

Seren's story is not unique. I believe this is the story of millions of children all over the world who are going through a similar situation. Children have no 'voice' – Seren certainly didn't have a voice. They don't have a voice about their education, their welfare, their safety, their fundamental human rights. We are so lucky in the Western world yet we have problems that are well documented – obesity, mental illness, and the overuse and incorrect diagnosis of millions of children with ADHD.

I can't stop or prevent Seren from taking medication when she gets older, but I hope she won't. I even heard her the other day slowing her breathing and trying to calm down, and then I overheard Karl say to her, 'Seren, are you ok? What do you need, how can I help?' She answered, 'Daddy, please can you get my oils and put my meditation music on'.

At that moment, I stopped and smiled and thanked the Universe. I thanked God and I closed my eyes and took a deep breath in and out, as in the moment I realised that I didn't save Seren, Seren saved herself.

I hope it helps

I don't know if Seren's story will help anyone. I hope it will. I hope it helps parents, but more importantly, I hope it rescues lots of beautiful little souls.

I hope it saves future children and generations to come. I hope it changes the way that parents, teachers, medical professionals, and our society treat hyperactive, spirited children. It might not do any of that; it might just get dusty on someone's bookshelf. Who knows?

If I have learnt anything throughout this whole journey, it's simply this: not to be afraid, to believe in myself and my child and my family. I must always believe that there can be a different way, that the experts don't always have the answers, and if I have faith that everything will be ok – so it will be.

I have learnt to fear less and love more.

The end

Epilogue

Today Seren is happy, really happy. She is loved, she feels safe, she feels secure, and now ADHD is only a positive thing in our family.

She doesn't have Oppositional Defiance Disorder anymore, and she no longer suffers from anxiety and low self-esteem.

However, this doesn't mean that as a family we will be happily sailing off into the sunset. Our journey is ever-changing and constantly moving as Seren is Seren, and her personality means that change affects her behaviour.

Life is one big, constant change, and this ride won't be for the faint-hearted. But it's our ride, our family and our journey, and we have finally learnt to live, love and laugh with it all.

Seren is doing better with her reading and writing, is playing the piano and has been selected to play violin in the orchestra at school. She is a talented gymnast and a great little artist, and we only have ADHD to thank for that!

A year ago, while she was on medication and seeing experts, this could only have been a dream, now it is a reality. If someone had told me that this incredible stuff would have happened to Seren, I would never have believed them. As a family, we were lost in the abyss; however, together with Seren leading the way, we followed the light and found home.

Albert Einstein, Walt Disney, Michael Phelps, Richard Branson, Michael Jordan, Jim Carrey, Justin Timberlake and Justin Beiber (one for the kids) all have one thing in common – they all have ADHD. All over the world it is seen as an illness, a disease, a disorder.

But can it be so terrible if some of the most talented and influential people on the planet have it? And how have they managed to survive and become the 'elite', if they all had this curse?

Do we want our future generations growing up feeling that they are flawed,
that their brains don't work correctly and that they need medication to function?

What message is this giving?

And where would we all be now if Einstein was medicated as a child?
Would the world look differently now?

And if Richard Branson had been labelled and told that he was different,
that his brain didn't work correctly, that he needed 'fixing', would the
Virgin global brand even exist?

Instead of thinking outside of the box, we need to get rid of the box! We need to throw the box away, in fact, we need to burn the goddamn box!

We need to come together as one, get rid of the stigma and start a positive ADHD movement. We need to support each other as parents and hold no judgments. We need to stand tall and realise that our children are not broken and they are not sick.

We could be holding the key to future creators, artists, musicians, entrepreneurs and world leaders (it is documented that Winston Churchill had ADHD).

We need to make our children brilliant again, because with love, respect and understanding, they could be the most amazing, awesome human beings!

I believe that it's our unique, high-energy, creative, risk-taking, fearless ADHD kids who can change the world.

Let's be the ones who help them do it!

References

1. The Columbian, 11 July 2016, Children with August birthdays are more likely to get ADHD diagnosis, viewed 29 November 2015, http://www.columbian.com/news/2016 / jul/11/children-with-august-birthdays-more-likely-to-get-adhd-diagnosis/

2. The Advertiser, 20 August 2008, Children misdiagnosed with ADHD, viewed 19 September 2016, http://www.adelaidenow.com.au/news/children-misdiagnosed-with-adhd/story-e6freo8c-1111117255077

3. Psychology Today, 8 March 2012, Why French Kids Don't Have ADHD, viewed 13 December 2015, https://www.psychologytoday.com/blog/suffer-the-children/201203 /why-french-kids-dont-have-adhd

4. Healthline, 4 September 2014, ADHD by the numbers: Facts, statistics and you, viewed 19 September 2016, http://www.healthline.com/health/adhd/facts-statistics -infographic#7

5. Australian Autism ADHD Foundation, 2014, Why the increase in Autism (ASD), ADHD and Neurodevelopment Disorders? viewed 22 March 2015, http://www .autism-adhd. org.au/why-is-adhd-increasing

6. The Telegraph, 10 March 2016, ADHD is vastly overdiagnosed and many children are just immature, say scientists, viewed 19 September 2016, http://www.telegraph. co.uk/ news/science/science-news/12189369/ADHD-is-vastly-overdiagnosed-and-many -children-are-just-immature-say-scientists.html

7. Virtual Medical Centre, 27 September 2009, Birth Statistics, viewed 17 September 2016, http://www.myvmc.com/pregnancy/birth-statistics/

8. Raconteur, 18 July 2013, Rising UK birth rate and increased demand for private care, viewed 20 September 2016, http://raconteur.net/healthcare/rising-uk-birth -rate-and-increased-demand-for-private-care

9. Australian Institute of Health and Welfare, 2014, Ceasarean Section, viewed 20 September 2016, http://www.aihw.gov.au/WorkArea/DownloadAsset.aspx?id=6012 954775

10. National Toxics Network, July 2010, A list of Australia's most dangerous pesti- cides 2010, viewed 19 April 2016, http://awsassets.wwf.org.au/downloads/fs025_a _list_of_australias_most_dangerous_pesticides_1jul10.pdf

11. Passmore, S 2014, The ADHD Handbook, Exisle Publishing, Australia.

12. Daily Telegraph, 14 December 2014, Surge in Ritalin use for toddlers 2-6, viewed 16 April 2016, http://www.dailytelegraph.com.au/news/nsw/surge-in-ritalin-use -for-toddlers-26/news-story/66c53f879e85c0487b5c8d1f3afc0fbd

13. The Atlantic, 7 July 2014, How Childhood Trauma Could Be Mistaken for ADHD, viewed 22 May 2016, http://www.theatlantic.com/health/archive/2014/07 / how-childhood-trauma-could-be-mistaken-for-adhd/373328/

14. Victoria State Government, Better Health Channel, January 2015, Naturopathy, viewed 22 May 2016, https://www.betterhealth.vic.gov.au/health/conditionsand- treatments/naturopathy

15. Natural Healthy Concepts, 27 May 2014, 5 Nutrients that can help kids labelled with ADHD, viewed 20 September 2016, http://blog.naturalhealthyconcepts. com/2014/05/27/adhd-nutrient-deficiencies/

16. Vogue Magazine, 1 August 2015, Dr Weaver, The Gut is created from the same tissue as the brain during foetal development, viewed 21 September 2016, http:// www.pressreader.com/australia/vogue-australia/20150801/282140700025987

17. Web MD, 17 December 2014, Study links low iron to ADHD, viewed 27 April 2016, http://www.webmd.com/add-adhd/childhood-adhd/news/20041217/study-links -low-iron-to-adhd

18. TEDx Talks, 10 November 2014, The surprisingly dramatic role of nutrition in mental health, viewed 10 May 2016, https://www.youtube.com/watch?v=3dqXHH- Cc5lA

19. Daily Mail, 10 January 2016, Shocking statistics reveal children as young as two are using antidepressants – and more than 26,000 under the age of 16 are being prescribed the medication, viewed 17 September 2016, http://www.dailymail.co.uk /news/article-3392290/Children-young-two-using-antidepressants.html

20. Breaking the Set, 8 May 2014, Why ADHD is Not a Disorder – Interview with Thom Hartmann, viewed 15 June 2016, https://www.youtube.com/watch?v- =yowurewU0qA

21. CBC News, 14 April 2014, Prisoners given powerful drugs off-label, allegedly to 'control behaviour', viewed 27 June 2016, http://www.cbc.ca/news/prisoners-given-powerful-drugs-off-label-allegedly-to-control-behaviour-1.2609940

22. The New York Times, 13 December 2014, The selling of Attention Deficit Disorder, viewed 30 September 2016, http://www.nytimes.com/2013/12/15/health / the-selling-of-attention-deficit-disorder.html?pagewanted=all&_r=0

23. ADDitude, 20 January 2012, Ritalin Redux, viewed 20 September 2016, http:// www.addditudemag.com/adhdblogs/11/9378.html

Acknowledgements

I would like thank my amazing publisher Lou Johnson for giving me the opportunity to share our story. None of this would have been possible without you and I will be eternally grateful for all your support and guidance. Thank you to my wonderful editors, Kit Carstairs and Michele Perry; for bringing the story to life and being so supportive throughout the process. Thank you to Alissa Dinallo for the beautiful cover design, Bronnie Joel Photography for the amazing photoshoot and to Jessica Twamley Hair Artistry. I have been so blessed to have worked with so many supportive, strong and empowering women who have each given me the confidence and strength to share our journey. And finally, thank you to Paul Carter for introducing me to Lou and for all the great advice along the way.

Endless thanks to my husband, Karl, for being there every step of the way with me. Like most guys, you didn't research anything on ADHD, and at times this would upset me, but I am truly grateful for you standing by me in my darkest hours. I love you with everything I have.

My beautiful parents, Bob and Karen, who spent hours on the phone, along with constant FaceTime chats when they were sick with worry (thank you, Steve Jobs). Karen, who spent hours and hours crying and researching ADHD, sending books from the UK to Australia, and moaning every time that they took three weeks to get here.

My best friend, Anna – even though you were 9,000 miles away, you were by my side always and I will be eternally grateful for this.

Our new friends in Australia that we met at such a vulnerable time, you will never know how much you saved us. Angie and Mike, what more can I say? Thank you Angie, for all the support, endless ADHD chats and for helping make sense of it all.

Daniel and Michele, thank you for all your advice and for listening to me harp on about ADHD every (like every) time I saw you.

Frankie, thank you for listening to me, supporting me and helping me through it.

To Pete and Marie, thank you. Pete, for inspiring me and making me realise that you can have ADHD and be awesome! And to your beautiful wife, Marie, thank you for being there for me and supporting us.

I didn't know one person with ADHD until I moved to Australia, and now some of the closest people to me have ADHD. If there was ever proof that the Universe or God, whichever you believe in, brings people to us, I know it's true because it happened to us.

And to Jade, our amazing babysitter, who at twenty-four has ADHD and has just finished studying to be a marine biologist. Thank you for being there for Seren when she had no-one, and I was at my wit's end! For riding bikes with Seren, climbing trees and picking shells, and for saving my sanity many, many times when you arrived at the door on a Sunday at 9.00 am, giving us all a few hours peace. I am so proud of you and I hope you are in our lives forever.

My brother-in-law, Billy, and his wife, Lucy, thank you from the bottom of my heart for everything – for listening, supporting us and being there for us.

And to Seren's teacher, Diane – the chats, phone calls and countless emails – thank you.

To my landlady, Ruth, in the UK, who became my long-distance counsellor, reading and responding to the monthly emails that I would send when I escaped to the hairdressers!

And lastly to my children – Seren, thank you for taking me to the lowest point that I have ever been as a mummy, but then holding my hand and rising again with me. We travelled the journey together and I so am grateful to you for being who you are, you have taught me so much. I love you more than you could ever know.

Finally to Daisy and Flynn, my little Tweedledum and Tweedledee. Daisy, thank you for being there for your baby brother, thank you for covering his eyes when Seren was having hysterical screaming outbursts, for teaching him the right way to do things and for being so grounded and calm at such a young age. I adore you and your beautiful spirit.

Flynn, thank you for being the coolest baby boy ever, you rock my world every day!

And not forgetting Chip, our faithful hairy friend, for letting me cry on you when I had no-one else to turn to. It has probably been a tough road for you too at times.

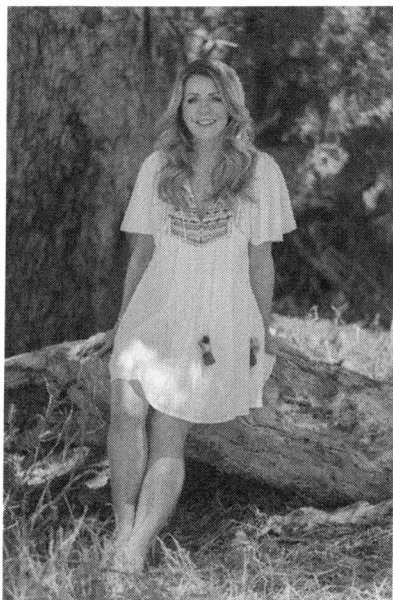

Susy O'Hare

Susy is an author, speaker, coach and ADHD mum. She is passionate about empowering parents to accept the child that they have and learn how to make peace with their child's differences.

Susy provides parents with an alternative, more holistic approach to parenting a child with ADHD. She empowers mothers to tap into their intuition, step out of a lens of fear, and parent through a lens of love.

Susy has driven the conversation around ADHD through public and social media to encourage parents to step into their power and discover how to help their child thrive. Through hosting talks and workshops in her community and providing online courses for her wider community, Susy has created a community of sisterhood where she shares weekly tips, tools and support for mums. She has featured as a guest writer for blogs such as Lifehack, Healthline and ADDitude magazine as well as being interviewed on various podcasts. Susy's journey has been featured in both local and national newspapers, magazines and mainstream television in Australia.

Susy is passionate about helping people to see that ADHD isn't a disorder, but just a different way to be. And that with the right tools and guidance - ADHD can be turned into a superpower!

Keep up to date with Susy at
www.susyohare.com

For more resources, help and support head to
www.diaryofanadhdmum.com

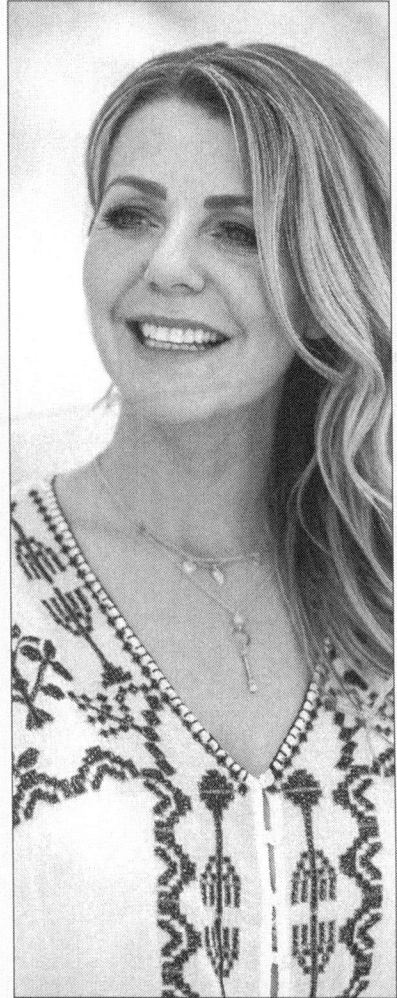

Manufactured by Amazon.ca
Bolton, ON